About the author

A former history teacher, Louis Proto has been exploring both eastern and western approaches to personal growth and healing for nearly twenty years. He led many awareness and bodywork groups both in Europe and America before going to India where he studied yoga and meditation for three years. Since returning to England he counsels for the Westminster Pastoral Foundation, has a private practice in London and runs training workshops in relaxation and Voice Dialogue. He is the author of *The Feeling Good Book*.

Also published by Century Arrow

The Bristol Diet *Dr Alec Forbes*
Curing PMT *Moira Carpenter*
The Long-life Heart *Arabella Melville*
Who's Afraid of Agoraphobia? *Alice Neville*
Overcoming the Menopause Naturally *Caroline Shreeve*

HOW TO BEAT FATIGUE

Put more zest in your life the natural way

LOUIS PROTO

Century Arrow
London Melbourne Auckland Johannesburg

A Century Arrow Book
Published by Arrow Books Limited
62–65 Chandos Place, London WC2N 4NW

An imprint of Century Hutchinson Ltd

London Melbourne Sydney Auckland
Johannesburg and agencies throughout
the world

First published 1986
Reprinted 1986

ISBN 0 09 946620 1

Set in 10/11pt Sabon
Phototypeset by Deltatype Lecru, Ellesmere Port, Cheshire
Printed and bound in Great Britain by
The Guernsey Press Co Ltd, Guernsey, Channel Islands

Contents

Acknowledgements

My thanks are due to the following:
Gail Rebuck, Publishing Director of Century Hutchinson, for suggesting the final chapter outline; Gabrielle Pinto for technical assistance with the sections on homoeopathy and acupuncture; Brian Butler for allowing me to include the Emotional Stress Release Technique from *Touch For Health* (Applied Kinesiology); the Dr Edward Bach Centre for permission to list the Bach Flower Remedies; Robert O'Dea for his kind assistance with the preparation of the manuscript for publication, and for the illustrations; my friends with whom I have shared over the last fifteen years the ideas contained in this book and to whom it is dedicated, with love.

Foreword

This book is about you and your energy – how you can handle it to stay healthy, positive and full of vitality and how you can bring yourself down and end up tense, drained and, possibly, ill. As well as showing you what to do when that happens, it is intended as a manual of self-nourishment and is ultimately about the *quality* of life.

CHAPTER ONE

Everybody's Problem: Fatigue

Anne is in her late forties, married and still considered an attractive woman. More often than not these days, though, when she looks in a mirror she worries about how haggard she's getting. Life is one long, mad rush from morning till night and she's just about had enough. Preparing breakfast for four people, getting herself off to her part-time job as a silver-service waitress, calling in at the supermarket on her way home, cooking again . . . She is getting to the point where she is sick of the sight of food. And when she staggers home loaded with shopping, the last thing she needs is an old lady clamouring for attention, but her mother has been living with them for several years now. She is not an invalid and, though arthritic, is mobile and likes to help her daughter when she can. But she has been alone in the house all day and wants a bit of company, whereas after a day spent at everyone's beck and call — fetching, carrying, travelling — all Anne wants is to kick off her shoes, sit down and take it easy before the others come home expecting to be fed. And she says so. Her mother retires hurt to her room, Anne feels guilty and sooner or later goes in to make things all right again. More pleasing other people and still no time for herself . . . Anne's husband has been working overtime recently as they are both saving up for a holiday in Thailand and their married daughter has agreed to have her grandmother for a few weeks then. It is really only the thought of that dream holiday that keeps Anne going — and early nights. Going to bed so early when her man is home late means they have little time together and Anne is secretly worried that her constant tiredness is having an effect on their love-life.

Harry is in the rag trade, and rich; he owns a big store on Oxford Street and smaller ones in the suburbs. For a former East

End barrow boy he has done very well for himself and attributes his success to hard work. He still drives himself hard although he no longer needs to, and doesn't trust *anybody* not to have their fingers in the till when he's not around. Harry is a difficult man to work for and just as bad to live with. Rachel, his wife, is in therapy and on tranquillizers, something he cannot understand at all. She has this lovely house, servants, money to buy anything she wants – and he is faithful. Not that he has any time or energy not to be, for after a day spent running his little empire he comes home feeling all-in. Conversation over dinner tends to consist of a monologue by Harry about his hassles during the day and the state of the economy. He eats a lot nonetheless and likes to end the meal with a Benedictine and a cigar (which Rachel loathes). Unless they have guests – more liqueurs, more cigars – the rest of the evening is usually spent in front of the television with Harry fast asleep, snoring. Rachel is seriously considering leaving her husband. The weekly sessions with her counsellor have made her aware how starved she is of contact, warmth, real sharing. Harry is too tired to give her what she needs any more and she is tired of living with him.

Debbie shares a flat in Streatham with two girl-friends and works in a trendy boutique on the King's Road, She came down from the provinces and finds London exciting, but sometimes a bit too much. The crowds and the traffic in the streets get her down most and the occasional difficult customer. It's a busy shop, with hi-energy disco played loudly all day to attract the predominantly young clientele. Lunch is usually coffee and a sandwich, fitted in between wandering in and out of shops and maybe queueing up at a bank to get some money. Food is not very important to Debbie. Neither she nor her flat-mates enjoy cooking, and anyway, she does not want to put on any more weight. When all three girls are in for the evening, they either eat what's in the 'fridge or share a takeaway if nobody has remembered to do the shopping, unless one of their boy-friends is coming round to dinner, in which case there will be a proper meal after which probably they will all go off to a disco. Debbie likes boys, dancing and staying out late, though recently she has been feeling washed out and has not been enjoying herself as much as usual. She finds it hard to get up in the mornings and has been warned at work about coming in late so often. Especially on Saturdays, she finds herself being too abrupt with customers and irritable with her friends after work. The disco music blaring relentlessly all day now grates on her nerves and sometimes she feels she will scream if they don't turn it down a bit. That journey backwards and forwards is getting her down too; it's more of a hassle every day, what with trains being cancelled and buses so often late. Perhaps she should change her job?

Like Anne, *Martin* feels under pressure and exhausted. For too long a teacher in the same school, he feels he is in a rut. After fifteen years of trying to teach history to totally unmotivated kids, he is disillusioned and as bored with his subject as they are with him. Having spent the day keeping order in the classroom, he flinches when he sees the piles of exercise books on his desk waiting to be marked. And there is more work waiting for him at home, since he works as an assistant examiner for a schools examination board to help pay maintenance to his wife from whom he is separated. No wonder he has started smoking again after having kicked the habit for six months. How on earth will he meet the deadline and mark 350 GCE scripts in three weeks, five essays to a script? He swears it is the last time he will let himself in for this sweat, money or no money. At home things are strained and he is not getting any support. His young daughter is staying with him and makes no secret of her resentment of Martin's live-in girl-friend. He feels caught between them, wanting them to get on together – and more and more fed up with the bitching and the sulks. At times, it is even a relief to escape upstairs to his room to mark scripts and let the two of them get on with it. But after burning the midnight oil too long his brain is so active that he lies awake for ages. He looks drained and feels it. He tells himself he should get a new job and a new lover – but lacks the courage.

John is a comfortably-off retired civil servant with too much time on his hands. His wife died last year and he is still grieving, though he never talks about her any more. A lot of the time he feels depressed, but tries to make the best of things and fill the day somehow. He feels loneliest at night as he lies in bed waiting, sometimes in vain, for sleep to come. More often than not, he does not feel refreshed when he wakes up in the mornings. Sometimes he is awake at dawn even though he did not get to sleep until the small hours. He has been to consult his doctor, who prescribed some pills which are either anti-depressants or tranquillizers – he is not sure. John wonders why he feels so tired most of the time, since he has so little to do. He worries about his health and is afraid of getting cancer like his wife. He keeps going back to see his GP, who has now written him off as a hypochondriac and has given up trying to reassure him about his stomach, bowel and prostate. The doctor's evening surgery is always full of people like John.

Fatigue is no respecter of persons – young or old, rich or poor, at some time in our lives we all fall prey to it. Some life-styles invite it more than others, but nobody escapes entirely. To feel tired at times is natural – after gardening perhaps, or following a strenuous game of tennis or squash. This type of fatigue we expect; it's not unpleasant and can be quite enjoyable. Indeed, provided the job has been well done (or we have won!) there is a certain satisfaction in relaxing afterwards, perhaps over a drink or in the bath.

The fatigue that we are considering, that we need to 'beat' – in the sense of learning how to handle and preferably forestall it – is unpleasant. It is insidious, devastating and, if chronic, potentially lethal. What we call fatigue is really shorthand for a wide range of states that include physical and mental exhaustion, depression, irritability, restlessness – in other words, generally feeling 'down' and unable to cope with the demands and pressures of our life-style. To be constantly fatigued affects the quality of our lives at every level. We experience our jobs as drudgery, drag ourselves to work in the mornings and can't wait until the day is over and we can go home again. The lack of ability to concentrate not only impairs our performance and our prospects, but could get us into real trouble. The miscalculations that may arise could be more serious than mere typing errors or those forgotten papers that made the boss so mad. The part played by fatigue in causing road crashes, for example, has been recognized by the government by way of legislation that empowers the police to make spot checks on the documents of lorry- and coach-drivers, to see if they are putting in too many hours' driving without a break. How many industrial accidents occur from the same cause is less easily checked, let alone how many hours' work are lost by absenteeism.

The more tired you are, the less desire you have to relate to other people. Anyone who has ever had to deal with the public – in travel, for example, or in the service industries – will know what a strain this can sometimes be. But if you are tired, it can be just *awful*; even a legitimate request feels like an intrusion. One of the hardest things to do when you are really drained is to be *nice* to people. This leads to problems in more intimate relationships too. Perhaps the biggest 'turn-off' is the partner who is always 'too tired' or, even worse, irritable. Fatigue and the consequent need to withdraw can be too easily interpreted as rejection, and the ensuing resentment can lead to rows or sulks. Alternatively, one partner may simply get bored with another who is never in the mood to play – and look elsewhere. Fatigue contributes to the break-up of more relationships than we realize.

Fatigue is also more of a health hazard than most people think. Persistent fatigue can be a symptom of many organic diseases and, if you continue to feel exhausted for too long, it is wise to go to your doctor for a thorough check-up. If, however, nothing shows up on your X-rays or in other tests, there is very little that a GP can do for you. For all its undoubted achievements, it is a sad fact that allopathic (i.e. 'straight') medicine has no cure for the physical and nervous exhaustion that hits every one of us from time to time. Palliatives, maybe, but remedies, no. It has been estimated that 40 million tranquillizers are taken each day and that over 20 per cent of the population in this country have taken them at some time or another in their lives. A vast number of these drugs together with anti-depressants are being prescribed by doctors; some of them are addictive, most have side-effects. To put it bluntly, when it comes to coping with fatigue, as with the common cold, you are on your own.

Fatigue, if persistent, is a warning signal that you are heading for trouble if you don't take a really hard look at your life-style. It should be taken seriously for, even if overt symptoms of illness have not appeared, it may herald them. For example, if Debbie does not start paying more attention to her diet and getting more sleep, her resistance will be lowered to such an extent that she is likely to succumb to any bug which happens to be around. If she is lucky, she may get off lightly with a cold or the 'flu; whether this develops into pneumonia depends on how strong her constitution is, but she's pushing her luck. Harry, at the rate he drives himself, over-eats, drinks and smokes is asking to be pole-axed by a massive coronary or a stroke. Anne and Martin, on the other hand – excessive worriers and under stress – are the types who end up with digestive ulcers, back trouble or what we used to call a 'nervous breakdown'. Unhappy, grieving John is a likely candidate for acute depression and possibly serious illness.

How then to beat fatigue *before* we fall ill or before it wrecks our work, relationships, peace of mind and capacity to enjoy life to the full? In the following chapters we consider alternatives to tranquillizers: ways to relax, ways of nourishing ourselves at all levels, ways to raise our energy-levels and restore quality to our lives.

CHAPTER TWO

What Causes Fatigue?

What exactly is this state which we use so many different expressions to describe? We can say, for example, that we are tired, worn out, frazzled, beat, on our last legs, a wreck or, if American, 'bushed'. The grosser amongst us will be 'knackered' (or something even more gross). There are as many ways of describing this Hydra as there are manifestations of it – aching muscles, lethargy, inability to relax or sleep, irritability, depression, anxiety, withdrawal and so on. Obviously fatigue is not just a physical state – it also affects us at mental, emotional and spiritual levels. Everybody knows that when they are ill they don't *feel* so good. If they have problems they can 'worry themselves sick', while if they become disillusioned and depressed they may feel 'tired of living'. The physical body and the thinking/feeling function are connected like a web: tap one part of it and repercussions will be felt along all the other strands.

High energy, Low energy

Body, mind and feelings, then, are all part of a continuum – **ourselves**. This continuum is constantly changing and is a dynamic energy-process. Human beings are receivers, transformers and transmitters of energy. We need energy merely to stay alive, let alone to move, to be active and creative. How much energy we have available varies from day to day, sometimes even from moment to moment. We recognize this fact when we greet each other. 'How are you today?' we ask, suggesting that you may not be the same as you were last time we met. What has changed? The short answer of course is, *everything*, not just clothes, make-up and hairstyle, but every cell in our body. But what we are actually inquiring about is the other person's health and mood, which is really the same as asking 'How is your energy today, high or low?' The person asked may well even reply that he or she is feeling 'low' or 'down', in which case you may try to cheer them 'up' and end by getting 'high' together. We often use the analogy of a battery in everyday speech when we say we feel 'recharged', 'drained', 'flat' or, on a really bad day, 'dead'. We are talking about our energy levels.

Kirlian photography has shown how our energy-levels and state of health are inextricably linked. A Russian electrician named Semyon Kirlian and his wife, Valentina, found a way to actually photograph the 'aura' of a person's energy field. Their invention consists of an aluminium plate to which a high-frequency field is delivered. This plate is covered by another plate of glass over which goes the film. The subject for the 'Kirlian effect' places his or her hand on the film, which is protected from salt in the skin by a piece of plastic. A pressure gauge ensures that the hand pressure is consistent. Using this technique, one ends up with the imprint of the subject's hand surrounded by patterns and colours – the energy-field. Kirlian found that when he was ill the energy-field photographed around his hand became blurred and faint, while that of his wife (who was well) remained clear and bright. Since then research has been undertaken in the USSR and, in the 1970s, in the West, and it has been shown it is possible to use Kirlian photography successfully for the diagnosis of certain disorders *before the symptoms become overt*. That there is a connection between low-energy states and 'dis-ease' – of whatever variety – is indisputable, as is the fact that our energy-levels change according to a definite rhythm.

According to the theory of biorhythms, there is a physical cycle of 23 days, an emotional cycle of 28 days and an intellectual cycle of 33 days. Each cycle when charted on a graph forms a wave-like pattern. On the days at the 'top' of the wave, energy in that sphere will be high and conversely, at the bottom of the wave it will be low. In between there is a critical period when energy will be unstable, especially if the critical periods of two or all three cycles happen to coincide. At such times the person will be especially prone to illness or accidents. The intellectual cycle affects concentration, judgement and the ability to learn. The emotional cycle affects moods and emotions, while the physical cycle affects body coordination and stamina. Biorhythms can be charted for each individual. The first biorhythm calculator was produced by the Swiss in 1927 and they have used them (as have the Japanese and the Americans) in factories for safety, in hospitals for calculating the best time to carry out surgery, and in the selection of national gymnastic teams for high-level performance.

There are times, then, when our energy-levels will be naturally high or low, quite independently of the kind of life we are living. It is estimated, for example, that 30 per cent of women suffer every month from premenstrual tension lasting up to a week or more. Other people are affected by the full moon and feel drained and unstable whenever it comes around. This is not really as far-fetched as it sounds when one bears in mind the effect of the moon's gravitational pull on the tides and the fact that so much of our bodies is water and the composition of our blood that of sea-water in particular. Gurdjieff said that the moon 'sucks' our energy and studies carried out at the University of Illinois on 100 patients over five years established that chest pains and bleeding ulcers were more frequent in two-thirds of the patients around the time of a full moon. There is not very much one can do about a full moon except be aware that one is likely to feel 'off' and make provision for that fact. However, there is now a great deal that can be done for premenstrual tension (Moira Carpenter, *Curing PMT The Drug-Free Way*, Century).

Moreover, there *is* much that we can do for the fatigue that we create ourselves by the way we live. Fatigue is a low-energy syndrome, so first of all we have to look at the reasons *why* we are so short of energy. If we use the analogy of the battery, then the reasons why we get fatigued become easier to grasp. We have simply 'run out of juice', either because we have made too many demands on our energy reserves or because we have failed to 'recharge' them sufficiently.

Are You Losing Energy?

'Losing' here means *wasting* energy, or losing it involuntarily. We don't necessarily lose energy every time we put it out. Sometimes the more we need, the more we get, just as muscles tend to become bigger the more we make use of them. It is like love: our store of love is not limited. The more capable we become of giving love, the more there is to give – and, hopefully, the more comes back to us. Athletes run marathons, mountaineers literally get high scaling peaks, tapping their reserves of endurance and stamina because they love what they are doing. If you really want to do something you will find the energy (and probably the money). Energy is mobilized by intention, and where there's a will there is always a way.

POOR MOTIVATION

However, one of the ways in which we lose energy is when we *have* to do things we don't want to do. When that happens the energy is not flowing naturally into the task in hand and so, in order to get it done, we have to make an effort and it is this effort that drains us. Furthermore, rather than just getting on with it, we may also resent having to do it, in which case it is just like trying to drive a car with the brakes on – not exactly a good way to get anywhere either fast or effortlessly! For many people, possibly even the majority, this is what their working life is about: not wanting to be there and making a chore of everything.

POOR ORGANIZATION

Even if you enjoy your job, if you are not well-organized you will put out more energy than you need to do. Having to hunt for a pen and a pad every time you want to take down a phone message, for example, is a drain, especially if you get irritated doing so. So is needing to check the same things over and over again because lists have not been kept, or running up and down stairs because you didn't work out in advance exactly everything you had to fetch. If you were to sit down and work out your own time and motion study, you would probably be amazed at the amount of energy you would save by planning, making lists and keeping things you use all the time in the same place so that they are handy when you need them.

OVER-COMMITMENT

Some people never have a moment to themselves when they can

'switch off' and relax. They are always 'on the go', either at work or socially. Their diaries are full of engagements, meetings, business lunches, dinner parties, bridge evenings and so forth. They set it up that way, either because they can't say 'No' or because they are 'hooked' on making money, having company or always being occupied. They end up with as little space for themselves as there is left in their diaries.

'OVERDOING IT'

If you complain to someone that you are feeling exhausted, they will probably advise you not to 'overdo it' – and they will be quite right. We 'overdo it' whenever we strain and put more effort into something than is really necessary, or do so at a time when we don't have the energy available to carry it out. There is a time to work and a time *not* to work – or at least to take a break for a while so that energy can accumulate again and we return refreshed to whatever it was we were doing. It has been found, for example, that most people can only concentrate fully for about an hour and a half, after which their attention starts to wander or they begin to make mistakes. These are signs that it is time to take a break and if we continue working we shall end up with all the symptoms of fatigue like eyestrain, stiffness and maybe a headache. With physical exertion it is even more essential to heed the warning signs of strain – pains in the chest and shortness of breath above all – otherwise we risk ending up with something much more serious than a headache. What drains us is going on beyond the point where, if we were more aware of our energy process, we would stop. This applies as much to playing as to working. Harry the workaholic and playgirl Debbie have much in common – and not only that they both feel 'wiped out'.

RUSHING

Having to work under pressure and rushing about drains us more quickly than almost anything else. It is really another form of overdoing things, for it requires us to put out more energy than we would need to do if we gave ourselves more time. Mostly we rush when there is no need. But this is not surprising since the whole way we live is geared to speed. Ours is the age of fast food, jet travel, instant everything from coffee to communications and entertainment. More and more gadgets come on the market every year, not so much to save us labour as to enable us to get more things done more quickly. Speed has become a value in itself, synonymous with efficiency. Not surprisingly, the sheer pace in our cities conditions us to rush without even being aware that we are doing so. It is only when one stops walking on a busy shopping street, maybe to look in a window, that one realizes just how fast everyone else is moving.

TENSION

Tension is not only a symptom of fatigue but also a cause – and almost certainly the *main* cause of so much of the fatigue experienced today. After all, in this day and age most people do not have to slave to earn a living. The people most likely to kill themselves with work or drive themselves to the point of collapse are those driven by ambition, greed or anxiety, so it is highly likely they were tense in the first place.

When we get tense, we start to lose energy. We drain ourselves on the physical level by stiffening up and holding our muscles tight, especially the belly muscles and the jaw, shoulders and lower back. Energy is wastefully expended in unnecessary movements, pacing up and down perhaps. If we are nervous we will probably talk compulsively, either to anyone who happens to be around or, if alone, to ourselves in our heads. The latter is called 'worrying'! It is hardly surprising that tension is the root of many of the classic symptoms of fatigue such as headache and backache.

Just as fatigue is caused by tension, so tension arises from stress; the more sensitive you are, the more the potential stressors in your life. These could include virtually anything: taking examinations, changing jobs, getting married, not getting married, moving house – even Christmas, a time dreaded by many lonely or isolated people. But even if you happen to be the most thick-skinned, easygoing or optimistic person, at times you will find yourself undergoing stress of some kind or another. It is part of the human condition and most of us manage to get through it either alone or with a little help from our friends, as the song goes. The real problem is *hidden* stress, stress that is in-built in our lives, that we take for granted and so do not realize that it makes us chronically tense.

STRESS

Broadly speaking, there are two types of stressors: those which assail us from the outside and those we generate within ourselves. The tension they occasion is, of course, always *within* us.

Outer stressors

The environment in our big cities is of itself stressful with its sheer pace, pollution, noise and over-stimulation. Much of our fatigue is caused by sensory overload and the result of long-standing over-stimulation of the sympathetic nerves. Assailed from all sides by a veritable bombardment of traffic sounds, petrol fumes, hoardings and posters shrieking for our attention during our working day – and maybe a noisy, crowded office as well – we return home to spend perhaps hours looking at more visual images on TV or being deafened by ultra-loud music at a disco. What with police and ambulance sirens, fire-engines, pneumatic drills, motor bikes and so forth, it is surprising that all city-dwellers did not go deaf long ago. Anything that hooks our attention but which is not of itself interesting drains us, for attention is energy. We lose energy, remember, by *having* to give energy in spite of ourselves and, with so much going on all around us so stridently, we have no choice but to look and listen *all the time*. Hence we become over-stimulated, sometimes to the point where we are so wound up that we find it hard to switch off, to relax and even to sleep.

But even those who are not exposed to the pressures of city life have to face the pressures to do with survival. For some, these will be about making ends meet in an age of recession and unemployment, or to do with keeping a business afloat. For others the stress may come from their own ill-health or that of a member of the family, or from sudden accidents. Life is never certain at the best of times and certainly not in this thermonuclear age, when the possibility of a global war worries many people sufficiently to make them want to march and otherwise demonstrate their anxiety to unresponsive governments. Fear of death is in-built into all of us, while bereavement and loss of love are the very greatest stressors of all.

Inner stressors
Dr Hans Selye was the first to point out thirty years ago in his trail-blazing work *Stress of Life* that the most dangerous stressors of all are those that come from within ourselves. Not only can they sap all our energy: they can make us physically and mentally ill, or desperate enough to kill either others or ourselves. People drive themselves mercilessly towards unrealistic goals, tear themselves apart with unresolved conflicts, torture themselves with phobias and inferiority feelings. Often they are their own worst enemies and judge themselves continuously and far more harshly than they would dream of judging others. Very few people are sure enough of their own worth and identity to love themselves unconditionally, putting their own health and peace of mind before the demands being made upon them from outside. Instead, they exhaust themselves trying to meet others' expectations or compensating for their own gnawing insecurity or sense of inadequacy. And so the world is full of perfectionists, workaholics, pleasers and people desperately trying to be what they are not – all of which takes up a lot of energy.

Holding on to negative feelings about others is draining too. These are usually related to fear or anger, powerful primary emotions which release adrenalin into the bloodstream to prepare the body for fight or flight. Often we do neither, but dither in a limbo of worry or resentment. Since the original threatening situation remains unresolved, the body muscles remain mobilized for defence or attack. When this is the case, the usual symptoms of tension will be manifested: fatigue, lack of concentration, irritability, restlessness, inability to relax or perhaps to sleep, aches and pains, lowered resistance and so forth.

Exposure to stress, especially over a long period, can drain our reserves of energy to the point where we may fall ill. Anyone recently bereaved or very depressed should be considered by those who care about them as being particularly at risk and needing to nourish themselves well. Let us ask ourselves now whether we too are doing this.

Are You Recharging Your Batteries?

We have said that human beings are receivers, transformers and transmitters of energy. Unless we are getting enough in the way of raw materials and processing them properly, obviously there will not be much to show in the way of the finished product – energy.

FRESH AIR

If we did not breathe at all, we would soon be dead. Oxygen is one of the basic raw materials of life, passed from the lungs via the red corpuscles of the blood to the muscles, there to be burnt to produce energy. If insufficient oxygen is getting into the blood, we may well feel jaded, listless and generally low on energy. This can happen when for any reason ventilation is poor. Every school-teacher knows that sometimes when the whole class is dozing off the quickest way to breathe fresh life into the lesson is to open a window. We associate yawning with fatigue and boredom, both low-energy states for which we attempt to compensate by drawing more air into the lungs. Concentrating on work becomes harder in a stuffy atmosphere, such as an office, simply because not enough oxygen is feeding the brain. Pollution in the air from traffic fumes or smoking has a similar affect. The absorption of oxygen into the blood is hindered by smoking, which also constricts blood vessels and thus affects the circulation of that oxygen. We may not be smokers, our home or place of work may be well-ventilated and still we may not be ventilating ourselves sufficiently because of shallow breathing.

FOOD

A major cause of fatigue is incorrect eating. We may be missing meals because we're slimming, too busy or just can't be bothered. We can get away with this for a while by drawing on our reserves, but soon the effects begin to show: we tire easily, become irritable quickly and begin to look as gaunt as we feel. But it is not a question of eating *more* so much as eating better quality food. Not all food is nourishing: junk food, for example, is usually high in calories (units of energy) but low in essential nutrients. The average man uses about 2,500 – 3,000 calories a day to convert into energy; the average woman approximately 1,750 – 2,250. A glance at this calorie count for common and not very nourishing foods reveals that it is not hard to make up one's calorie requirement:

FOOD	CALORIES PER 100 GRAMS
biscuits	400–500
chocolate	about 500
cream: single	200
double	460
doughnuts	355
ice cream	over 200
jelly	259
pastry	over 500
popcorn	482
potato crisps	550
shortbread	521
sugar	394

The last in this list, sugar, is virtually the only food that provides no nutrients whatever – which really makes it the junkiest of junk foods. And the most unavoidable too, for it is added to a wide range of supermarket items like soft drinks, certain kinds of pickles, some packet soup – indeed, it is hard to buy anything that *doesn't* contain sugar. Taking it in tea or coffee accounts for about 50 per cent of the average person's consumption of sugar, which is a staggering 110 lbs a year. This is hardly surprising, though, when you consider that one slice of chocolate cake contains the equivalent of ten and a half teaspoons of sugar! It would seem that many people are getting nearly a quarter of their calorie intake from sugar alone; the trouble with this is not only that their teeth decay and they put on weight – they also risk getting diabetes and coronary heart disease. And although sugar is an extremely concentrated form of energy, paradoxically if we have too much of it, after an initial 'buzz' we feel 'down'. Too many chocolates can leave us with 'sugar blues': the body responds to the sudden influx of sugar into the bloodstream by producing insulin, which lowers the blood sugar level too much. Since the brain can only use blood sugars as fuel, it starts running in low gear. The result is drowsiness, irritability and difficulty in concentration. And these effects are felt quickly because when we are inactive the brain is using quite a high percentage of our total energy consumption (about 500 calories a day).

The inadequacies of most modern diets are now being recognized by some governments. It has probably come as something of a shock to inhabitants of affluent societies to be informed that well-fed they may be, but well-nourished most of them certainly are not. The report of the National Advisory Committee on Nutrition Education (NACNE) on diet and health recommended cutting down the consumption of refined sugars, while the McGovern report suggested that this be halved. In the USA too, following reports naming sugar, salt, saccharin and junk foods as the cause of premature deaths, compulsory food labelling for contents and ingredients was brought in as early as the 1970s. Disturbingly, it was found that on the average supermarket shelves were products which contained a total of 608 toxic additives. It has been estimated that in England the average person gets through 6–10 lbs of additives per year, many of which have never even been tested for toxicity. It is not known exactly how many chemicals are added to food in order to make it look or taste better and last longer – perhaps around the 3,500 mark! Eric Millstone, lecturer in Science Studies at Sussex University, suggests that anyone addicted to junk food may be consuming anything up to 30 lbs of additives over a year. Since 1962, the EEC has issued directives on additives and those permitted in most member countries have been given a number preceded by an 'E'. The main categories go roughly like this:

E 100 on	mainly colourings
E 200 ,,	,, preservatives
E 300 and E 321	antioxidants
E 300 on and 400 on	mainly emulsifiers and stabilizers

But many additives used in this country have been banned by other members of the EEC and, if they appear on labels at all, do so just as numbers, though this is due to be changed in 1986 when the name also will have to appear. The most well-known additive is monosodium glutamate, responsible for the so-called 'Chinese restaurant syndrome'. Those allergic to this additive can react with dizziness, palpitations, headaches and nausea.

We may be allergic not only to the additives used in food

products but to food itself, even nutritious food. Pioneered by Dr Theron Randolph in the USA in the 1950s, research into food allergies is now becoming increasingly respectable in Britain too. Experiments carried out, for example, at Cambridge and at the Middlesex and Great Ormond Street Hospitals in London have established the connection between food allergies and a whole range of 'dis-ease' including arthritis, hyperactivity, eczema and so forth. One man's meat literally can be 'another man's poison'. An allergy to virtually any food could be behind fatigue, severe weakness, hyperactivity, backache, headache and depression. In America it has been estimated that no fewer than half the cases of depression could have a food allergy as their cause.

It is essential to eat the right food. But it is just as important that we assimilate it properly for it to nourish us. We may be *over-eating* – like Harry, the wealthy businessman – in which case we put so much strain on our digestions that there is little energy left for anything else, quite apart from the fact that we may get fat and thus have more weight to drag around with us. It may be too that we eat at the wrong times, when it is harder for the body to process the food adequately – just before retiring for the night, for example, or when we are tired or upset. Constipation can make us feel as sluggish as our bowel, so can fatty foods (and drinks) that affect the liver.

It is not only our bodies that need the right nourishment. Our mind, heart and spirit also need refreshment if we are not to be dull, bored, jaded, depressed and arid. Later chapters consider ways to get out of any rut in which we are dragging, to re-awaken our zest for life and, with luck, to experience the joy of living. But first we must start with basics: how to recharge our batteries and how to avoid losing energy.

CHAPTER THREE

Self-nourishment

IS THIS YOU?
'I never take a lunch-break – we all just send out for sandwiches.'
'After a working day, I'm usually so whacked I pick up a take-away.'
'I can't be bothered to cook for myself when I'm alone. It's not worth the bother.'

DO YOU BELIEVE THAT
Unless a meal is hot and contains meat, it is not a 'square meal'?
Vegetables are boring?
Raw food is for rabbits?
You will die (or at least faint) if you fast for a day?
Coke is 'the real thing'?

DO YOU LIKE
Sweets, chocolate, cakes and sticky buns?
Coffee black and strong – and lots of it?
Chips with everything?

If your answers are all or mostly 'Yes' then you are very probably not getting enough nourishment. Self-nourishment is about eating the right food, correctly prepared and correctly digested.

What is the 'Right food'?

Proteins, fats, carbohydrates, vitamins and minerals according to your daily requirement. If you feel 'run down', easily tired or low on energy, then you are most likely to be short of protein and vitamins.

PROTEINS

Proteins are the building bricks of the body and the stuff from which all our cells are made. Throughout our lives we need to take in protein for growth and repair; it is also a source of energy. We could manage without protein in our diet for a few weeks if necessary, relying on our reserves in the muscles. But soon the effects of protein deficiency would make themselves felt: lack of energy, inability to concentrate, low blood pressure, anaemia, low resistance to infection and fatigue due to the retention of waste fluids in the tissues.

The amount of protein you should be eating will vary according to your energy output, but a safe guideline for most people would be 1½ oz (40 grams) a day and about 25 per cent of what you eat. If, however, you are undergoing stress, are pregnant or convalescing, you will need more. These are the main foods which contain protein:

meat	nuts
fish	bread
eggs	pulses
milk	fruit
cheese	vegetables
poultry	

It will be seen from the above list that there are animal proteins and vegetable proteins. We need a mixture of both. Some of these foods are higher in protein content than others in the list, as will be seen from the following:

FOOD	PORTION IN OZ	PROTEIN IN GMS
beef (lean)	4	30
cod	6	30
chicken	4	33
egg	1 egg	7
milk	1 glass	6
cheese	4	28
nuts (brazil)	4	32
bread	3 slices	10
beans (baked)	4	7
banana	4	1
apple	4	0.4
carrots	2	0.4
cabbage	4	0.8

It should be easy to check whether you have been getting enough protein in the course of the day or merely stuffing yourself with more calories. Remember that during or after an illness more demands are made on your system and protein breakdown is speeded up, so you should take more at these times.

Since it will be readily apparent from the list of protein content above that vegetables and fruits are not in themselves adequate suppliers, vegetarians should be particularly careful to ensure that they are getting enough protein, especially if they are vegans. Beans and pulses, if eaten together with whole grains, will provide an adequate supply. Soya is an especially good source of protein and, as tofu, is one of the world's most popular sources of high-quality, low-cost protein, especially in South-East Asia. Tofu also has the advantage of being entirely free of cholesterol and very high in polyunsaturated fats – and it only contains 52.6 calories per 100 grams.

Whether or not you object to meat on aesthetic grounds, purely on health grounds it is advisable to eat less of it. This is because:

1 Flesh foods contain sodium salts which tend to make the blood acid. A slightly alkaline blood stream is needed for good health.
2 Meat is hard to digest and causes putrefaction in the bowel. Toxins could be absorbed via the colon and this could possibly contribute to cancer of the bowel, the second commonest form of cancer in Britain.
3 The blood of slaughtered animals often contains antibiotics and other drugs which have been administered to prevent or combat disease.
4 Animal fat, in which meat is rich, is conducive to heart disease, the world's biggest killer today.

FATS

Fats provide energy, too much of it: ounce for ounce, twice as much as sugar or pure protein. The problem here is not that we may not be getting enough, but that we are almost certainly getting too much – and of the wrong kind. Some fat in the diet is necessary, because it contains essential acids which are part of tissue-structure and help in the regulation of blood clotting. But we *need* only a small amount of fat – about 30 grams or 1 oz per day – whereas we eat probably about four times as much as this. As in the case of sugar, fat doesn't always *look* like fat and is present in disguise in many foods. However lean joints look, meat always contains a lot of fat, as do sausages, bacon, salami, hamburgers and meat pies. According to a National Food Survey in 1983, meat and meat products accounted for over a quarter of the fat consumed in the average British diet. Milk, cream and cheese made up nearly another fifth, while the contribution of pure fats – oils, butter, margarines, lard – was just over one-third. We tend to forget that fat is also used in the making of biscuits, cakes and pastries. The danger of eating too much fat is not simply that we *get* fat, but that we may have a heart attack.

Both the National Advisory Committee on Nutrition Education (NACNE) and the Committee on Medical Aspects of Food Policy (COMA) have recommended that we cut down on fats. The latter of these (unfortunately-named) bodies has spelled out why:

'Comparisons between countries have shown a strong positive relationship between the proportion of dietary energy derived from saturated fatty acids and mortality from coronary heart disease.'

The cholesterol in saturated (animal) fats that causes arteries to clog up and clots to form may not be the only culprit in causing an estimated one in three men to have a heart attack during his working life: other factors such as stress, smoking and lack of exercise also contribute. But it does mean that we should cut down on meat, eggs, butter, hard cheeses, milk and cream and go rather for fish, low-fat cheeses, soft vegetable margarines, yoghurt, skimmed milk, whole grains and cereals, vegetables and fresh fruit. It also means that we should trim fat off meat before eating it, grill rather than fry and drain fatty foods. Of the fat that we eat, a higher proportion should be polyunsaturated.

CARBOHYDRATES

The term 'carbohydrate' refers to both sugars and starches and the vital distinction we have to make is between processed and unprocessed. Unprocessed starches – whole grains, for example – are digested slowly, for it takes time for the layers of fibre to be broken down. As a result the sugars which are produced – all starches are broken down into sugars in the process of digestion – are released slowly into the bloodstream. But with refined sugar and processed starches the bloodstream is immediately flooded with sugar and we have seen the effect this has: irritability, drowsiness and the inability to concentrate. Even worse, not only have refined starches been stripped of their fibre, they have also lost most of their nutrients in the processing.

Carbohydrates make up pretty well 50 per cent of the calories in the average British diet, mostly in refined starches and sugars: white bread, biscuits, cakes, confectionery and breakfast cereals. Instead of these, we should be eating more nuts, seeds, whole grains, wholemeal bread and flour, beans, peas, pulses, vegetables and fruit. Not only are these more natural time-release energy capsules, they are also rich in vitamins, minerals and fibre.

Although bread has been one of mankind's staple foods for thousands of years, today buying our daily bread can be a confusing business because there are so many different types of loaves to choose from. For the reasons we have already outlined, it is better to avoid white bread – however delicious those crusty baguettes look! Go rather for the bread that has more of the wheatgrain and the fibre and is therefore better for you. 'Brown bread' used to be the term applied to all types of bread made from brown flour, but it is inaccurate since each flour is different. What is labelled 'brown bread' nowadays is in fact bread which has had 10–15 per cent of the wheatgrain removed during milling and now contains only half the fibre of flour which has had nothing removed.

Wheatgerm breads
Made from brown flour to which about 10 per cent wheatgerm has been added, which contains B and E vitamins and about 1½ grams of fibre per large slice.

Wholemeal breads
Made from flour that contains *all* the wheat grain and so has lost nothing of the natural goodness, especially if it has been stoneground by the traditional method of crushing the grain between two large millstones. Since all the outer part of the grain

is intact, wholemeal bread is coarser than other breads and contains more fibre – 4 large slices provides about 11 gms. It is obviously unnecessary to 'fortify' wholemeal bread with vitamins and minerals as these are present naturally. Since the Second World War, white bread has been thus fortified with thiamin, niacin, iron and calcium.

Granary or malted mixed grain breads

Made from brown flour to which have been added crushed wheat and rye grains, together with malted whole wheat. These breads are nuttier in flavour than other breads, darker in colour and keep longer because they are moister.

VITAMINS

Vitamins are so called because they are vital – for health, well-being, life itself. Whenever we are feeling 'under the weather', 'run down', fatigued or depressed, we need to check first whether our bodies are getting enough of these chemical substances which they need but cannot make for themselves. So this is *our* daily responsibility – and not a heavy one, since the total vitamin intake we need each day amounts to less than 100 milligrams (about 1/280th of an ounce).

All the vitamins are needed to maintain the functions of the body and to feel good. But for our purposes – the avoidance and correction of fatigue – the B vitamins in particular are crucial and we shall be considering them in detail. First, however, make sure you are getting enough of the others from the right foods which contain them. In the following sections, RDA = recommended daily intake; the vitamin content in food is measured by international units (iu) or, in capsule or tablet form, by micrograms (mcg). 1 mcg = 3.33 iu.

Vitamin A (also known as retinol and carotene)

Essential for growth, health of eyes, bones, skin; keeps lining of lungs, throat, digestive and reproductive systems in good order.
RDA: 1000 mcg (3,300 iu).
Natural sources: liver, green leafy vegetables (spinach, parsley, cabbage, salads), red and yellow fruits (apricots, melons, rose-

hips, oranges). Carrots are especially rich in carotene (one carrot provides nearly seven times the RDA), so is liver (4 oz provides nearly six times the RDA). The richest of all sources of vitamin A are halibut and cod liver oil.

Signs of deficiency: poor night vision, pimples on arms and legs, flaky skin, catarrhal and bronchial infections.

Vitamin C (also known as ascorbic acid)

Necessary for healthy gums, teeth, bones, skin and blood vessels. Essential for forming healthy connective tissue and also promotes healing. It is now known that this vitamin, together with vitamins A and E, strengthens the immune system; they are therefore likely to protect against cancer and, possibly, AIDS.

RDA: variously estimated from a minimum of 30 mg upwards. Some authorities suggest that for high resistance to infection and optimum well-being, doses should be at saturation level. Since this vitamin is water-soluble it cannot be stored in the body, so we cannot overdose on it as may happen with the fat-soluble vitamins A, D, E and K.

Natural sources: fresh citrus fruits, rose-hips, blackcurrants, strawberries, tomatoes, green and leafy vegetables, green and red peppers, potatoes.

Signs of deficiency: low resistance to infection, slow healing, sore gums.

Vitamin D (D, D2, D3)

Needed to ensure the proper intake of calcium and phosphorus by the bones and teeth.

RDA: 100 iu

Natural sources: fish liver oils, sardines, salmon, herrings, eggs, butter, margarine, sunshine on skin.

Signs of deficiency: weak, twitching muscles; tooth decay; retarded or crooked bone growth.

Vitamin E

Assists the supply of oxygen to the heart and muscles. Essential for the integrity of the red blood cells. Acts as an antioxidant for polyunsaturated fatty acids in tissue fats. Protects other nutrients from oxidation.

RDA: Estimated at 10 mg. (1 mg = 1.36 iu)

Natural resources: seeds and nuts, wheatgerm, cold pressed vegetable oils (e.g. sunflower oil), green leafy vegetables, whole grain cereals, eggs. One 4 oz serving of muesli provides half the RDA, while the same amount of spinach supplies a quarter of the RDA.

Signs of deficiency: poor skin, muscle cramps, early ageing. This vitamin is associated with many good things like maintaining youth, combating pollution, improving one's sex life and easing premenstrual tension!

Vitamin K

Essential for blood clotting.

RDA: Not known

Natural sources: liver, green vegetables, soya beans, oils.

Signs of deficiency: prolonged bleeding from cuts or wounds.

THE NERVE AND ENERGY VITAMIN

Any book dealing with the problems of fatigue and tension must direct special attention to the necessity of keeping up levels of vitamin B. This is because most of the B vitamins are concerned with the ability of the body to convert the food we eat into energy, and also because they are essential for maintaining the nervous system. Folic acid and B12 are especially needed for the production of red blood cells, so a deficiency could cause serious anaemia. Since the B vitamins are water-soluble they cannot be stored in the body and therefore have to be supplied every day. They merit a separate section, simply because they are the most complex of all the vitamins.

B1 (thiamin)

Essential for growth, health of muscles and nerves and the conversion of carbohydrates into energy.

RDA: 1.4 mg

Natural sources: meat, fatty fish, beans, nuts, seafood, whole grains, pulses, potatoes, wheatgerm, yeast. Six slices of wholemeal bread supply half the RDA and 4 oz of steamed broccoli supply two-thirds.

Signs of deficiency: fatigue, irritability, depression, neurotic disorders, loss of appetite, poor digestion.

B2 (riboflavin)

Extracts energy from proteins and carbohydrates. Essential for growth, health of skin, eyes and red blood cells and for general well-being.

RDA: 1.6 mg

Natural sources: meat, soya beans, eggs, vegetables, poultry, milk, cheese, yeast, wheatgerm. One pint of skimmed milk provides two-thirds of RDA and 4 oz of mackerel provides one third. Since this vitamin is destroyed by sunlight, don't leave your milk out on the doorstep!

Signs of deficiency: lack of stamina, nervousness, dry hair and skin.

B3 (niacin, nicotinic acid)

Essential for growth, digestion of carbohydrates and health of nervous system and skin.

RDA: 18 mg

Natural sources: lean meat, whole grains, fatty fish, poultry, nuts, dried fruit, potatoes.

Signs of deficiency: headaches, insomnia, irritability and, in extreme cases, schizophrenia.

B6 (pyridoxine)

Essential for the body's use of protein and the health of nerves, skin and muscles. Helps to maintain good circulation and to prevent heart disease.

RDA: 2 mg

Natural sources: meat, fish, whole grains, poultry, green vegetables, milk, oats, fruit (especially dried). One large banana supplies a third of daily needs, 6 slices of wholemeal bread about a quarter.

Signs of deficiency: irritability, shakiness, insomnia, depression, anxiety.

Folic acid (folate)

Essential for all growth, healthy blood and fertility.

RDA: 400 mcg

Natural sources: spinach, endive, Brussels sprouts, broccoli, whole wheat flour, lentils, potatoes. A 6 oz portion of the latter provides half the RDA, while 4 oz of lentils supply a quarter.
Signs of deficiency: anaemia, weakness, fatigue, depression.

Biotin
Needed for healthy nerves, skin and muscles.
RDA: 1 mcg
Natural sources: liver, kidney, eggs, nuts, bran, wheatgerm.
Signs of deficiency: eczema, loss of hair.

Pantothenic acid (B5)
Extracts energy from proteins, fats and carbohydrates.
RDA: 4–7 mg
Natural sources: no particular foods, but most foods do contain some.
Signs of deficiency: Dry skin and hair.

B12 (cobalamin)
Essential for the body's use of protein and for health of nerves, blood and skin.
RDA: 3 mcg
Natural sources: liver, poultry, lean meat, eggs, yeast, miso.
Signs of deficiency: fatigue, anaemia.

VITAMIN DEFICIENCY
The lists above provide handy references to check, both for possible vitamin deficiencies and for foods which will repair the lack. But there are times when it may be necessary to take vitamin supplements as well. It is well-known that large doses of vitamin C taken at the initial onset of a cold may be effective in aborting it. Also that it could be good to take cod or halibut liver oil capsules in the winter months when there is little sunshine around to stock us up with vitamin D. Not so well-known perhaps are the following examples of times when taking extra vitamins has been proved to be advisable:

- when you are ill or convalescent
- if you are a heavy smoker or drinker

- if you have to rely on institutional catering (including hospitals!)
- if you are slimming
- if you are under stress
- if you are using contraceptive pills
- if you are pregnant
- if you suffer from premenstrual tension
- if you are on antibiotics, diuretics (e.g. for high blood pressure) or indeed any synthetic medicines, even aspirin.

Vitamin A is the one of which you are least likely to need more; indeed, you should be careful not to overdose on it. If you think you are deficient, eat some liver or munch a few carrots. The ones to watch are vitamin B and C. A study carried out at St Mary's Hospital, Paddington showed a connection between vitamin B6 deficiency and depression for some women on oral contraceptives, and suggested that up to 50 mg of this vitamin a day would be effective in changing their mood. Other tests at St Thomas' Hospital, London proved that 50 mg of the same vitamin taken for a fortnight before the commencement of their period partially or totally relieved premenstrual tension in seven out of ten women. In the first months of pregnancy extra amounts of folic acid are necessary, and this vitamin should also be taken by heavy drinkers – and the boozers amongst us should also make sure they have extra B1, since this is the first one to go. Because vitamin B12 is found only in animal foods vegetarians, especially if vegan, should also make provision for getting it from another source. If you smoke, drink or are on the contraceptive pill (or all three, plenty of foods rich in vitamin C should be eaten, as this fragile vitamin is destroyed by all three in the body. Also, large doses – 500–1000 mg daily – should be taken when convalescing, especially after surgery.

MINERAL DEFICIENCY

It is also possible that fatigue may be due not to vitamin but to mineral deficiency, especially of calcium or iron. Minerals cannot be manufactured by the body, but are present in the soil as inorganic elements. They are absorbed by plants, which may in turn be eaten by animals, so we get our supply from a variety of plant and animal foods. The body needs more than fifteen different minerals for health, growth and energy and deficiency in some of these can result in fatigue, depression, emotional tension or anaemia.

Calcium

There is considerably more calcium than any other mineral in the body, 99 per cent of which forms the skeleton and teeth. The remaining 1 per cent is circulated round the body in the blood and is essential for muscle contraction, functioning of the nervous system and blood clotting. A deficiency of calcium seriously disturbs the function of muscles and nerve cells, with the result that we are excitable, unable to relax or sleep properly. The daily requirement is 500 mg, more for young people and pregnant or nursing women. The main natural sources of calcium are dairy produce, fish, vegetables and eggs.

Iron

Iron's best-known function is its use as a part of haemoglobin ('haem' in fact means iron), the carrier of oxygen from the lungs to every cell in the body. A deficiency of iron therefore starves the cells of oxygen and this could be the cause of feeling under the weather, tired, irritable and depressed. It is one of the causes of anaemia, which in medical language simply means a shortage of iron. Iron-deficiency anaemia has been recognized by the Department of Health as being very common in this country, especially among women. Those who have really heavy blood loss during periods may need to take iron supplements to compensate. The RDA for men is 10 mg, for women it is 12 mg (the US RDA is 18 mg). Foods rich in iron are dark meat, liver, kidneys, dried apricots, prunes, wholegrain cereals (muesli and Weetabix are specially rich), spinach, lentils and peanut butter.

You are unlikely to be deficient in other minerals if your diet is good. Phosphorus, magnesium, sodium, potassium and sulphur, for example, are present in most foods, especially proteins, and if you include whole grains, green leafy vegetables and an occasional portion of liver you cannot go far wrong.

It may be necessary, however, to take mineral supplements if there is an increase in the body's normal requirements, e.g. during pregnancy, after an operation and during illness. Phosphorous and magnesium deficiencies are rare, as these occur so widely in foods, but can arise when, for example large magnesium loss is caused by alcoholism or chronic diarrhoea. Similarly, potassium and sodium are so widely distributed that it is almost impossible not to get enough. The following gives some idea of where these minerals are found and what they are used for by the body.

Phosphorus	Foods rich in calcium and protein. Teeth and bone structure. Energy storage and transmission.
Magnesium	In most foods, especially vegetables. Important for energy transmission.
Sodium	In most foods, especially table salt. For muscle contraction and conduction of nerve impulses. Keeps body fluid environment constant.
Potassium	In most foods, especially fruit, fruit juices and cereals. As for sodium.
Sulphur	In all protein foods, e.g. meat, fish, eggs, milk, cereals. Used for building body protein and connective tissue. Active blood purifier.

VITAMIN AND MINERAL LOSS

You may have chosen the right foods, but unless they are properly prepared the nutrients they contain will not get to you. We have seen that vegetables provide a very high proportion of the vitamins and minerals we need in our daily diet, but these can be lost in the process of cooking, especially Vitamins B and C which are soluble in water. They are also partially destroyed by heat, and Vitamin C can be destroyed when cut surfaces of foods are left exposed to air. For this reason, quite apart from the fact that they make delicious salads with the right dressings, vegetables should be eaten raw at least some of the time; in that way all their goodness is preserved, our teeth and gums get exercise and so does our digestive system because of the valuable fibre. When you do cook vegetables, avoid vitamin and mineral loss by remembering the following tips:

- If possible, either do not peel them or peel very thinly (or scrape carrots, for example). Much of the goodness is concentrated just under the skin, which is itself fibre.

- Do not leave washed, peeled vegetables lying around for hours. Even worse is to leave them soaking in water.
- Cut pieces of vegetables into small pieces, using a sharp knife. In this way you prevent crushing or bruising and cut down on cooking time.
- Either cook in very little water, or save the water and use for stocks. Steaming is the best way to cook most vegetables. Chinese-style wooden steamers with lids can be placed on top of saucepans already cooking away – and that saves on your fuel bill too!
- Fast stir-frying seals in vitamins and makes a delicious meal. Use as little oil as possible and preferably buy yourself a wok. If you like, you can add a little water to the stir-fry and finish them off by steaming gently.

Either avoid using salt altogether, or use it very sparingly. Salt is bad for health – or rather, if we take too much it helps its friend cholesterol to clog up arteries and hence produce a stroke or a coronary. Remember that the salt you add to your food is only one-third of your total intake: it is also present in many other foods you eat, such as animal products, cereals and processed foods. Flavour with soya sauce or tamari instead – it's better for you.

Right Digestion

Selecting the right foods and preparing them correctly are essential, but unless your body processes them properly you might just as well have eaten junk for all the good they will do you. More tips:

- After working, give yourself time to unwind before you tuck in.
- Do not eat if you are angry or otherwise upset. Do not cook either if you are in this frame of mind: even if you don't cut or scald yourself, you will turn out a meal at best tasteless or at worst toxic.
- Eat SLOWLY. The digestive process starts in the mouth – so

chew food thoroughly before it reaches the stomach.
- For preference, do not drink *during* a meal as this dilutes the gastric juices, although it is hard to refrain when lunching or dining with friends and, say, sharing a bottle of wine. However, when eating alone try having your drink *after* the meal.
- Do not eat too late before going to bed at night.
- Do not eat too much. Come away from the table feeling satisfied but not bloated.
- Every so often, give your stomach a rest. Going without food for a day occasionally will do no harm. However, make sure you drink plenty of water or juice while you are fasting, and choose a day off work when you don't have to put out a lot of energy. If during a working day you are too pushed to take a lunch-break – and this should not be allowed to happen to often – it is better to miss eating altogether for once rather than to grab at any junk that happens to come into the office. Turn deprivation into an opportunity to fast – and eat well later!

FIBRE

For thousands of years yogis have believed that disease is the result of toxins released into the blood from food residues in the large intestine: in other words people eat the wrong food and then do not properly eliminate what is left. Certainly if we are constipated, we don't feel exactly on top of the world. On the contrary, we feel headachy, fatigued, irritable, literally 'uptight'. Our modern Western medicine recently seems to have validated the ancient insights by drawing attention to the need to clear out the bowel thoroughly, so as to avoid not only constipation but also diverticulosis, piles or worse. The best way to do this is by including more fibre in the diet.

Not only does roughage in the form of fibre prevent constipation and reduce the risk of digestive disorders; it also helps to reduce the absorption of fat and to slow down the absorption of sugar. We should consume about 1 oz of fibre each day (25–30 gms), but in fact only get on average ½–¾ oz (15–20 gms). Denis Burkitt, a surgeon who was one of the first to urge us to take more fibre, has an embarrassingly simple test to see whether we are following his advice. 'Are you', he asks, 'when you go to the "loo", a "large floater" or a "small sinker"?' Mr Burkitt approves of large floaters.

Where can we get more fibre from? Wheat bran is the best-known form and bran cereals flood the breakfast-food shelves nowadays in the supermarkets. But other foods can supply our requirements too, if we know their fibre content. A loaf of wholemeal bread, for example, contains about 1 oz of fibre per pound as compared with a similar loaf of white bread which has only about ⅓ oz. Here are a few more foods to compare for fibre content:

CEREALS	QUANTITY	DIETARY FIBRE IN GRAMS
Unprocessed bran	2 tablespoons	9
Bran breakfast cereal	6 ,,	8
Wheat breakfast cereal	2 pieces	6
Wholemeal bread	1 slice	4
Porridge	6 spoons	2
Cornflakes	3 ,,	1
VEGETABLES		
Baked beans	4 tablespoons	7
Lentils	2 ,,	3
Sweetcorn	3 ,,	3
Potatoes	} 1 medium-size portion	2
Cauliflower		2
Lettuce	6 leaves	1
FRUITS		
Banana	1 medium size	4
Apple	1 ,, ,,	2
Orange	1 ,, ,,	2
Pineapple	1 thick slice	2
Grapefruit	half	under 1

CLEANSING DIETS

Occasionally the liver as well as the bowel needs to be detoxified, especially if we have been indulging in alcohol and rich foods or eating too much fatty or fried food. Signs that this needs to be done are irritability and feeling 'down', lack of energy and perhaps a bloated feeling under the rib-cage. Also, in Chinese medicine the classic indication of liver malfunction is the marked presence of frown lines between the eyes, while puffiness and bags *under* the eyes mean that the kidneys are being overloaded. If these signs are present simultaneously, it really is time you went 'on the wagon'! But sharing alcohol is so embedded in our Western culture as a form of togetherness that it is hard sometimes to say 'No' to a drink without the risk of being thought unsociable. It's only when you may have decided to do this that you realize how it all adds up – a sherry before dinner, wine with the meal, perhaps a pint or two at the local. Alcohol is a tricky issue from the point of view of relaxation: a drink after work certainly help us to unwind and fosters conviviality, since people feel less tense in each others' company. But it does build up in the liver, affects moods and energy levels and ultimately acts as a depressant.

The commonest cleansing diets are based on limiting intake to foods which can detoxify and at the same time provide adequate nourishment, while drinking plenty of non-stimulating fluids. Fruit, vegetables, brown rice and potatoes do the trick, the last two having the added advantage of absorbing toxins from the bowel on their way through the digestive system. Here are some diets you could try to see which suit you best.

How long you stay on any of the diets is up to you and will depend on your commitments and stamina, but should not be too long – suggested periods are given in each case. It would be inadvisable to go on a diet at all if you are pregnant, breast-feeding or engaged in work which demands a lot of energy or which is stressful. Expect to feel occasional giddiness or head-aches: this is due to the toxins being released into the bloodstream on their way to being flushed out of the body and is a sign that the diet is cleansing the tissues. If it is quite impossible for you to go on a full cleansing diet, what you could do is just be very careful what you *do* eat. Strictly avoid junk foods, alcohol, sugar and coffee; leave out meat, fish, poultry, eggs, cheese and all dairy foods (which create mucus) for a while, until you feel clearer and 'lighter' again.

Grape fast: Not more than three days.

About 4 lbs (2 kg) should last the day. Eat the skins as well and chew the pips. Do not attempt this diet without your doctor's approval.

Fruits or fruit juices: One day in every month will give your digestion a rest, purify the blood and leave you feeling clean and clear-headed.

Oranges, apples, grapefruit or pineapple according to preference. Raw juices have no equal for keeping an alkaline balance of the blood; they also contain lots of vitamin C which is a powerful blood detoxifier.

Raw vegetables and vegetable juices: One week to ten days' duration. Remember to take vitamin B supplements (the whole complex or Brewer's yeast with added B12).

Carrot juice is particularly good. As well as being delicious, it contains nearly all the vitamins and minerals required by the body. In salads remember to include watercress, a powerful intestinal cleanser and blood purifier which is rich in iron and iodine. Also fresh parsley, which is rich in iron as well as vitamins A, B, C (very much so) and E. Remember to choose the freshest vegetables and to use a sharp knife when chopping and slicing them. Use fresh lemon juice with a little oil (NO salt!) for the dressing and include as much garlic as you can take. Garlic has long been known as a natural antibiotic and cleanser of both the digestive tract and the blood. If you are expecting to spend an intimate evening with friends, then you might feel more comfortable taking your garlic in the form of capsules which can be bought at health food stores. Onion is good for our purposes too, especially as onion soup – but eat the cooked onions as well as the liquid.

Potatoes: Two to three days should be enough to clear you out.

Prepare them in any way you like except fried or sautéed – in other words, no oil. Eat the skins as well and if you have boiled them, save and drink the water. Do not add butter.

Brown rice: A week to ten days is the classic macrobiotic cleansing diet.

The technique of cooking this is to work it so that the rice is ready to eat just as the last of the water is absorbed. It depends

whether you like your rice chewy or soft, but a safe ratio would be
2½ cups of cold water added to 1 cup of rice. Cover the saucepan
with a lid, bring the water to the boil, then turn the heat right
down and allow to simmer until the rice is cooked. When most of
the liquid has disappeared, test for chewiness. If it's ready, take off
the lid and allow the rest of the water to evaporate; if still too raw,
add a *little* more water. You could try adding seaweed to the
water, or preparing the seaweed and adding it separately to the
cooked rice. (Dried seaweed in various forms is sold in health food
stores; the Japanese use it a lot and it is very rich in minerals,
especially iodine.) If you find the cooked rice too bland, flavour it
with soy sauce or, better, tamari.

Drinks

It is important to drink a lot while on a cleansing diet, but avoid
alcohol, tea and coffee. Instead drink water (preferably mineral
water), fruit juices and herb teas. Of the latter rose-hip (very high
in vitamin C), camomile and mint are particularly good. Lemon
and honey form a good combination, and can be taken first thing
in the morning with a spoonful of cider vinegar.

TONICS AND 'PICK-ME-UPS'

The effect of a cleansing diet will be felt gradually. But sometimes
we are feeling so run-down, shattered or under pressure that we
need something to raise our energy, without the backlash likely
from sugar or caffeine. Chemists and health food stores offer a
bewildering array of proprietary 'tonics' that promise to do the
job. Maybe they do, maybe they don't, but invariably what they
all have in common is that they are expensive, while some are full
of chemicals and some are faddy. Multivitamins are hit-and-miss
and usually woefully low in potency on the very vitamins you may
need in massive doses. If you are irritable or fatigued, the vitamin
most likely to be deficient is one of the B complex, and the danger
here is that by overdosing on just one of them, you can cause a
deficiency of the others. However, here are some suggestions
which should not produce any problems.

Brewer's yeast

Brewer's yeast contains all the B vitamins except B12. It is 36 per
cent protein, with almost no fat, and contains fourteen minerals.

The most natural way of topping up on your intake of the vitamin most necessary for staying on an even keel, it comes either in powder form or as tablets. Since it has a strong flavour, the best way to take the powder is in orange juice – one tablespoon a day is enough.

Ginseng
This interesting root has enjoyed recognition as a medicinal plant for over 4,000 years in the Far East, where it is called 'the root of life'. Chinese doctors still prescribe it today for loss of vigour (including sexual potency), anaemia, nervous disorders and insomnia. It has such a powerful effect that it should not be taken late in the day, since it can stop you from sleeping. The Russians apparently give ginseng to their astronauts on space missions in order to heighten their alertness, energy and endurance – so it should be effective in getting you through the rigours of your working day too! The plant grows only in a few dry and mountainous areas of the world and the best quality ginseng comes from Korea. Ginseng takes six to seven years before it reaches maturity when the roots can be harvested, which is why it is so expensive. But it is such an energy-booster, so rich in nutrients, minerals and trace elements that it is worth the cost. Ginseng is marketed in various forms: the root itself, as tea, or in vitamin-like capsules of varying potency.

High protein drink
Another pick-me-up, which also serves to counteract cholesterol by adding lecithin, is made as follows.

Ingredients: *1 tablespoon lecithin*
              1½   ,,   protein powder
              1   ,,   wheatgerm
              1 glass milk
              honey (to taste)
              fruit of your choice
Mix in a liquidizer, chill – and enjoy.

Calcium supplements
When feeling strained and unable to cope, try boosting your

calcium intake with calcium lactate over a short period: it is obtainable from high street chemists, usually in 300 mg strength, the dosage marked on the bottle. Calcium pantothenate is also effective when under stress.

CHAPTER FOUR

Slowing Down

DO YOU SOMETIMES FEEL:
So wound up and restless that you can't sit still, let alone relax?
Kept wide awake by the thoughts rushing round in your head?
That your work is getting on top of you?
That you never seem to have time for yourself?
That you never seem to have time for *anything*?
At a loss whenever you have nothing to do?
Guilty when you take it easy?

If so, then it is high time you learnt to slow down before you give
yourself a heart attack. We all live under enough pressure as it is
without adding to it ourselves by unnecessary effort, rushing and
compulsive activity. Two things are necessary before you can even
start to relax and they are: giving yourself *time* and giving yourself
space.

Taking Your Time

It is easy to get into the habit of rushing, even when there is no
need. As we have noted, everything in our modern Western
society is so geared to speed that it has become almost a value in
itself. All around us things move fast: traffic, crowds, news. It is
not surprising that we ourselves become caught up in this frenetic
activity and perhaps even fear that we shall be left behind, miss
something if we are not 'in the swim'. We may be the types who,
like Harry in the rag trade, wear ourselves out in the rat-race to be
successful, or, like Martin the teacher, in order to make more
money 'on the side'. For them, time is money and time off is losing

money – or at least not making it. Debbie-types are also prisoners of time in a different way. Their philosophy is rather: 'Life is short, so let's make the most of it.' But working or playing too hard is the same in terms of energy loss – and life may turn out to be even shorter than we thought. Moreover, going too fast even defeats the object. Quite apart from the possibility of accidents or falling ill through overdoing it (which means that you can't do them anyway) the experiences of both work and play are diminished by the tension and the fatigue that ensue. Harry may indeed be a dull man as a result of all work and no play; he is also a very tired man – and, as for Debbie, she's a wreck!

DON'T OVER-STRUCTURE

Martin, at least, has got the message that some things are worth more than money – and the *quality* of your life is one of them. Next time you are offered extra work or social invitations, before you accept check on commitments you have already undertaken. Remember that what looks quite innocent and manageable in the diary may turn out to take up a great deal of energy in actual fact in terms of travelling, for example, or getting home late. It is always easier to say, 'No' when first invited to do something than to say, 'I'm sorry but . . .' and let someone down at the last moment when you find that you have taken on too much. There is also the possibility that you might miss out on some unexpected fun simply because the friend you haven't seen for ages happens to fly into London for a day – or that country cottage is yours for the weekend if you'll feed the cats – and you're unavailable. There is no use sulking while struggling to finish the work you have promised will be ready by Monday, or sitting bored out of your mind at Auntie Flo's dinner table – it's too late! Be more flexible with programming your future. As far as possible, make things provisional and only commit yourself definitely when it is absolutely necessary. Be cautious with your promises to be anywhere at any time – but once made, try to keep them. It is better to be thought hard to pin down than considered unreliable.

GIVE YOURSELF TIME

Be especially wary about committing yourself to time schedules; wherever possible, leave it open. After all, anything can happen to the best-laid plans of mice, men and women: the project could turn out to be more time-consuming than at first thought, or there might be unexpected demands on your attention which have to be dealt with straight away. Pressures there will always be: just don't add to them unnecessarily. If necessary, it is better to court displeasure by asking for more time than to kill yourself trying to meet unrealistic deadlines. After all, if you do have a coronary it will be yours, not theirs! Try to space out your times of concentration and effort so as to coincide with the periods in the day when you are naturally at your most alert, for you will get more done in a shorter time than when your energy is low. For some people this will be early in the morning, when others are still struggling to surface and face the world. Immediately after meals is a natural low-energy time for most people, understandably so since energy is going into digestion. Better to take a nap, go for a walk, or at least work on more routine matters at low ebb times than to strain your concentration.

Don't concentrate for too long at a stretch and be alert to the warning signals that it is time to take a break. Ignoring these signals is asking for fatigue, eyestrain, stiff neck and muscles and the possibility of over-stimulation to the point of insomnia. One person I know regularly gets a rectal abscess each time he has to wrestle with a backlog of work – clear proof that he finds it more than just a pain in the neck! It could just as well be a cold sore or a stomach upset or headaches – all protests from the body that it is being placed under stress and drained of vital energy. Breaks need not be long, for what is really needed is a relaxation of concentration. Just to stand and stretch – maybe a visit to the washroom if you are tied to a desk, or a tea-break – anything to refresh the brain a little. And often new ideas will surface during the time away from the work in hand, for the subconscious will continue working even when we are not consciously doing so. Agatha Christie used to say that her best plots came to her while she was doing the washing-up, while Archimedes' principle, as every schoolboy knows, surfaced in the bath-tub. It is a common experience that the best way to recall something to mind is to stop calling it: when we relax, it comes of its own accord. Often the best way to deal with a problem when completely stuck is to let it go, sleep on it and allow the subconscious to process the data by itself. The model of the atom on which atomic physics is based reputedly came to Niels Bohr in a dream, as did 'The Rite of Spring' to Stravinsky. By giving yourself such breaks (in every sense) you may not be wasting time but in fact *giving* time for your creativity to surface. During such breaks avoid coffee, because this will make you even more 'speedy'. Tea contains caffeine also, but you would have to drink twenty cups of it to match the 'buzz' that one coffee gives. Incidentally, the condition called 'jet-lag' can be minimized by drinking water during a long flight instead of alcohol. This is because after four hours in the air the body starts to dehydrate, a process accelerated by drinking alcohol. Taking a bottle of mineral water on board with you would probably be kinder to the cabin crew than summoning them for your water every hour.

CUT OUT UNNECESSARY EFFORT
Rushing takes effort and puts strain on all systems in the body, including the respiratory, vascular, digestive, muscular and nervous systems. In other words, we become out of breath, constipated or the reverse, fatigued and uptight. Move fast when you have to – but *only* when you have to. Whenever you catch yourself rushing from one place to another, pause and ask yourself: 'Am I in a hurry?' – and if not, slow down. Nine times out of ten you won't be, for rushing becomes a habit with all of us. Even if you are, 'make haste slowly' as the Latin proverb goes. Shifting from foot to foot at the bus stop, straining your eyes into the distance and cursing the bus company will not make the bus materialize any quicker, but it will leave *you* fatigued and irritable. All unnecessary movements such as fidgeting, drumming your fingers and pacing up and down are simply ways of losing energy. So is all unnecessary talking – one of the sure-fire ways of getting drained very quickly, especially if you are merely being polite.

Paradoxically, effort sometimes gets in the way of performance. Obviously the acquisition of technique is a prerequisite for mastery in any field and, in the beginning at least, sustained effort and practice is necessary to acquire it. But once the technique is there you don't have to kill yourself to come up to scratch: the best performances are those that appear relaxed, easy, flowing. It is the concentration and not the effort that makes the virtuosity of a Rubinstein or of Torvill and Dean. The grace with which they weave their arabesques, the ease of those horribly difficult leaps (whether up the keyboard or into the air) – this is what brings an audience to its feet with applause. It is possible to *relax* into action rather than to push and strain. To quote Christopher Dean after winning an Olympic Gold, it is like 'a sort of hypnotic trance, in which all the work you have done before comes out of you'. If you can't roller-skate, let alone ice-skate, and 'Chopsticks' is the only piece in your repertoire, still you can try to cultivate effortlessness in whatever activity you happen to be engaged upon. Whether or not the result will be any better, at least *you* will certainly feel better – and probably live longer. If you are still in doubt that 'easy' can sometimes be 'right', consider the mess the centipede would get into if it *tried* to move each leg instead of just walking. Whatever it is you are doing, relax into it, just 'do it'. Don't lose energy by adding to what needs to be done needless haste, worry and effort.

Taking Your Space

Just as we get fatigued from overdoing it and rushing about, so we become drained of energy if exposed for too long to outside stimuli. At work we may well have our statutory 40 square feet of space, yet still feel hemmed in by the people around us or plagued by distracting noise and comings and goings when trying to concentrate. It is not surprising that a link has been established between aggressive behaviour and overcrowding. We all need to withdraw from time to time into our own space and recharge our batteries if we are not to feel drained and irritable. This applies as much to the home as to the work environment; happy, and rare, are the families which respect each other's space as well as their togetherness. Possibly many rows are simply the result of over-exposure to each other, and occasional absence may indeed make the heart grow fonder. But nobody ever *gives* anybody their space; we have to take it for ourselves.

PHYSICAL SPACE

Probably very few of us are courageous enough to take our space when we need it. It feels somehow selfish or aggressive to withdraw attention from others we are with, especially if we love them. Also they may resent us, or feel threatened by our 'switching off'. Yet recognizing and allowing the spaces between friends helps to keep relationships fresh, for you know that when you spend time together it is because you really want to be together and not just a matter of habit. Also you are more likely to enjoy each other's company if your energy is high than if it is low – and the best way to generate high energy is to spend some time on your own, just taking it easy. If you are with people who don't know you well and might consider you unsociable, take your leave with grace when you have had enough small talk, perhaps looking at your watch and murmuring something about another engagement – but *don't* stay out of politeness and then complain afterwards that they never stopped talking. It's always up to you to take the space you need when you start to get tired – and this doesn't have to be done aggressively.

Sometimes of course it is not possible to withdraw totally and to relax in the way you would like. But you can always give yourself a breathing space. We have seen how the body naturally produces a yawn when it feels low on energy. Here are some breathing exercises which will freshen you up whenever you are feeling jaded and listless.

1   Close the right nostril with the right thumb. Inhale through the left nostril to a count of four. Hold the breath for a count of four.

2   Let go of the right nostril and close the left nostril with the left index finger. Exhale through the right nostril to a count of four. Breathing should be gentle and unforced.

3   With left nostril closed, inhale through the right nostril to a count of four.

4   Right nostril closed with the right thumb, remove the index finger from the left nostril, hold breath for a count of four and then exhale through the left nostril.

5   Repeat the whole sequence a few times only.

1 Place the hands behind the back in a comfortable position, the back of the right hand in the palm of the left hand, thumbs crossed. Relax the shoulders and jaw, allowing them to sag.

2 Breathe in deeply and slowly through the mouth to a count of four. Hold for a count of two. Exhale to a count of four. Rest for a count of four.

3 Repeat the whole sequence for as many times as feels good. Don't force the breathing, rather let it happen. The chest remains motionless throughout, only the ribs expand and contract, accordian-fashion. If you experience hyperventilation in the form of dizziness or tingling fingers, stop immediately and breathe normally.

1 Breathe into the belly. When you begin to feel bloated continue breathing, but higher, into the area around the stomach.

2 Now breathe into the chest until the lungs are filled up. *Don't force.*

3 Hold, then exhale from the upper chest down to the belly. Total inhalation should be to a count of five; hold for three; exhale to five.

A breathing exercise that cleanses and recharges (although it may startle anyone else who happens to be near you) is the 'Bellows Breath'. Simply breathe in and out rapidly through the nostrils, keeping the mouth closed. Do this to a count of 10 – then relax.

As well as filling our blood with oxygen, these breathing exercises are real mood changers when we are upset, tranquillizers when we feel het-up, energy-chargers when we are depleted. Our breathing patterns are very much connected to our energy-states. Novels abound with characters who pant with desire, gasp in astonishment, sniff with disdain or snort in disgust. The reader may well put down such a novel with a sigh of relief. Shallow, fast breathing goes with 'nerves' and tension, while holding the breath completely is a sign of intense expectation or fear. When we are relaxed, contented or asleep, our breathing pattern slows down and deepens. Strangely enough, we can create the mood by getting into the breathing pattern that goes with that mood. Try this for yourself. By breathing fast and shallow, you may well actually start to feel anxious, for example. We can use this to create a relaxed mood by slowing down and deepening our breathing pattern.

Just as changing your breathing pattern can change your state of mind and move your energy, so changing body posture could help to make you feel less tense. When our energy contracts, so do our bodies. We hunch our shoulders, tighten up muscles, hold in the belly. We frown and may clench our teeth as well as our fists. If we find the environment threatening we will probably sub-consciously protect vital organs by folding our arms across the chest and maybe crossing our legs. Unlocking this tight posture will make us feel more relaxed and literally 'expansive'. Stretch, breathe deeply as if you feel you really *belong* in this world and are entitled to any space you may take up in it. Then, when you sit down again, settle into the sort of open posture that you would naturally slip into if you *were* feeling contented and relaxed. Make yourself *comfortable* and take up as much space as feels good. Often you can get to feeling good by acting *as if* you were already feeling fine rather than waiting – perhaps in vain – for the OK feeling to come by itself without any prompting. We shall be exploring this further when we come to discuss autogenics in chapter five.

It certainly is a big help to slow down if surroundings are restful. There are few things more soothing than to walk in the countryside, surrounded by open green space under the vast sky and amidst the sounds of Nature. Alas, not all of us can escape into the country at the first signs of tension and 'inner city blues', though some of us are fortunate enough to have gardens or to live near parks. But we *can* always bring Nature into our living space to remind us that another world, green and pleasant, awaits us out there whenever we can make the time to go and enjoy it. Indoor plants, window-boxes – perhaps even posters of mountain scenes or tropical, palm-fringed beaches – these can be a sight for sore eyes, as can a softly-lit aquarium with beautiful little fish swimming lazily through the stones, reeds and bubbles. Lighting and judicious choice of colour are important too in creating a relaxing atmosphere in which to unwind more easily. Indirect lighting is always preferable to direct light, except for working by, in which case the light should fall on the page (or whatever you are working on) rather than shine into your eyes. The atmosphere created by placing night-lights or candles strategically around a room can be quite magical, as well as restful. As regards colour, green is the most soothing of all colours which is probably why it is so much used in hospitals, operating theatres and so on. Combined with white, green is the best colour to choose when decorating a room that is to be used primarily for relaxing. Blue is relaxing too, though somewhat cold. Reds are too stimulating, blacks depressing for most people.

PSYCHOLOGICAL SPACE

You may have taken your physical space, withdrawn from company, given yourself days off and so forth – and *still* feel under pressure. The body may have given itself time off, but the mind has not. In the East the mind is seen as a monkey, chattering incessantly, leaping from branch to branch, never still. Minds are always thinking, planning, worrying, finding us things that 'need' to be done, brooding on the past or fantasizing – usually apprehensively – about the future. Getting psychological space means giving your mind a rest, slowing down its mad chattering and shelving, at east for a while, all its pressures on you to 'do'. This, you may well be thinking, is easier said than done. True: it takes discipline to break the habit of compulsive thinking and that discipline is called meditation. It is a technique that can be learned and, if practised regularly, restores to us our freedom of choice as to which of the thoughts which come welling up are worth thinking *about*. Meditation gives us a psychological breathing space: it centres us when we are scattered and frenetic, slows us down, heightens awareness of priorities in our lives and where we are really at and mobilizes the nervous energy needed to accomplish our goals. From being harassed victims of pressure to get things done, we start to experience what it is like to initiate and be creative, to respond rather than simple to react. This makes all the difference in the world to the quality of life. It is the difference, say, between having to rush to get somewhere we are supposed to be, as distinct from simply deciding to take a walk in the park because it's a nice day.

MEDITATION

In religious traditions of both East and West meditation is a path to transcendental states, union, enlightenment, self-realization – call it what you will. But in recent years meditation in various forms has come to be practised by many people in the West because it is so effective in helping us to switch off the pressure and to relax. Research has proved that meditating reduces hypertension and produces changes in heart-rate, skin conductivity and respiration. In its best-known form of transcendental meditation, it has been adopted by business corporations in America as conducive to more efficiency and smoother interpersonal relationships within the organization.

Meditation can be done anywhere, at any time. Really, it is not 'done' at all, but happens when we *stop* 'doing'. We are not trying to get anywhere or to achieve anything when we meditate; we have already had too much of these activities. Being go-getters, achievers, doers is precisely the problem we want to correct by meditating – to make any kind of effort here would make the whole thing just another chore, something else we have to do. The Japanese call meditation 'zazen', 'just sitting', letting the world go by – the outside world of sounds and the world of inner sounds (thoughts) also. It is a 'non-doing', a 'just-relaxing', a 'just-watching' - like sitting on the top deck of a bus looking out of a window, happening to notice this or that without being particularly interested one way or another. Similarly, don't be particularly interested in any thoughts, feelings or body sensations that come while you are sitting in meditation – just observe them all impartially as if they were shoppers passing you on the high street. The same with noises from the outside, traffic, transistors, planes passing overhead and so on – just let them be there. For nothing is a distraction when you don't have a goal. And for meditation to *be* meditation, there must be no goal; you just sit because you want to sit and whatever happens while you are sitting is what happens. There is nowhere you have to get because you are there already – and that's a relief. Or, to change the metaphor, since you just came for the ride wherever you end up is OK.

Sometimes it can be a bumpy ride, especially when you first start meditating. You may feel fidgety and restless, your thoughts racing and convinced that you are wasting time. It may not be comfortable at first, but it is positive in that you see for yourself *why* you are so frenetic, for this is what is going on with you all the time. You *are* restless, thinking compulsively all the while and afraid of wasting time. But now you are aware of it and not *acting* from that space and wearing yourself out. 'So what, I still feel just as tense sitting like a dummy as when I'm rushing around like a maniac', may be your reaction to being asked to sit quietly doing nothing for a while each day. Maybe you will at first – but simply by watching and experiencing this tension, this compulsion to do, by not acting it out, by not feeding it, by and by energy starts to go out of it and you begin to feel more relaxed, calmer, under less pressure. Outside the periods of meditation you will begin to slow down, to take things more easily, not to push yourself so hard – or at least you will know now when you are not giving yourself psychological space.

So fasten your seat-belt and let your meditation take you wherever it wants to take you. Be passive for a change but also alert, watching with indifference the whole succession of body sensations, feelings and thoughts that will arise. Let the body relax but stay aware, thus reversing the usual everyday state of bodily tension and relative unawareness of our own process. It is like being wide awake in a body that is sleeping, but don't force attention or *concentrate*: just be a watcher. Adopt a position that facilitates this attitude, that enables you to relax into the body without falling asleep. The traditional posture for meditation is sitting on a firm cushion or two with legs crossed tailor-fashion – or, if you can do it, with one foot on the other thigh sole-upward, the other foot tucked under the other thigh in the 'half-lotus' – but sitting on a chair is almost as good. If you do choose to sit on a chair, the feet should be on the floor and the back should not be leaning against the back of the chair. Get comfortable, keep the back straight without straining, close your eyes. The hands may be either joined loosely together in any way that feels right, or resting lightly on the thighs, preferably with palms uppermost. If sitting on the cushion becomes uncomfortable after a while, shift into a kneeling position with buttocks resting on the heels, with or without the cushion for extra support.

For your regular meditation sessions, choose a quiet place in the house. Turn down the lighting so that the light is subdued (but the room is not dark) or light a few candles. Burning a stick of incense can help to sweeten the vibrations, as can having flowers within view. It is good to keep to the same time of the day for your sessions if possible and also to meditate in the same room. This regularity and familiarity of the surroundings will make it easier for you to slip into a calmer space sooner. Also, meditating regularly in the same room creates a peaceful vibration and whenever you come into the room you will feel it if you are sensitive. It is easier to relax into a meditative space if you are not afraid of being disturbed, so it is good to arrange, for example, not to receive phone calls or otherwise be disturbed during the time you will be meditating. Don't eat before a meditation session, or drink coffee or alcohol. If you have just come home from work or have been rushing around allow time to 'come down' before sitting. Remember that the art of meditation was first developed in monasteries and ashrams (Eastern spiritual communities seeking self-realization under the guidance of a Master). Their serene atmosphere was and is far less busy than the market-place in which we live.

Sitting quietly, doing nothing, the unwinding process will start to happen if you allow it. In fact, the only way you can stop it from happening is to interfere with it by *thinking* rather than *watching* thoughts come and go. In order to avoid getting 'hooked' by any worries, you may have to decide beforehand that you are going to shelve them for a while and not try to solve any problems until later. This time is time for yourself just to *be*, to relax into yourself. If, however, the 'monkey' mind is really hyperactive, the following tips should prove helpful.

Counting the breaths
Breathe normally, but after each exhalation silently register a 'one', 'two' and so on. Count after each exhalation up to 'ten' and then start again. If you lose it and get trapped into following a train of thought, go back and start again at 'one'.

Feeling the hara
The 'hara' is the part of the belly just under the navel. It is our centre of gravity and the source or channel of vital energies. While sitting, let your attention focus on the hara and really feel it. If

attention wanders into thoughts or outside distractions, keep bringing it back to this part of the body.

Holding a mantra

A mantra is a word or phrase charged with energy for us which, repeated continuously, has a calming and centring effect on the mind. Choose to repeat to yourself something evocative of relaxation like 'Slow Down', 'Easy, easy', or simply 'Relax'. Feel as if you are holding the mantra in the hara region and listen carefully to the word as you say it to yourself.

The length of your meditation sessions is up to you. Don't give up too soon because your mind is still driving you crazy – you may as well put up with it while sitting on a cushion as let it push you into hyperactivity which will use up more energy. On the other hand, don't persist for too long beyond the point where to sit for any longer feels like being greedy or forcing it. Once you have glimpsed the possibilities of serenity, inner stillness and freedom from pressure offered by meditation, you will start to look forward to having time to be with yourself for a while each day. Meditation refreshes you, slows you down and recharges your batteries.

The fruits of meditation will stay with you longer if you don't throw them away by falling back into bad habits of losing energy by rushing around, talking more than is necessary and putting out more effort than is necessary. Try to stay meditative throughout the day. What does this mean? Even if you have a resistance to actually sitting down and meditating, you can still receive some of the benefits by practising aspects of meditative practice. These include:

> awareness of the body
> stillness
> keeping energy in
> present-centredness
> no goals

We shall be discussing the all-important matter of body-awareness in the next chapter on techniques for relaxing the body. Already we have suggested that we lose energy whenever we fidget and move around involuntarily. So whenever there is nothing you *have* to do, don't do anything! Just relax, make yourself comfortable and allow the energy to gradually build up again.

Learn to enjoy those moments when you are alone as well as when you are with people. Value silence as well as communication, for silence is rapidly becoming a rare experience in this noisy world and it refreshes the spirit. Whenever you are feeling swamped by the mass of input from outside – in big stores or crowded trains for example – practise keeping your energy in so as to avoid getting drained. We put out a lot of energy through our eyes, so only *look* when you want to see something in particular. Otherwise keep the eyes unfocused – what used to be called in monastic circles 'custody of the eyes'. If you catch yourself being pulled out by the chaos around you, breathe into the hara to centre yourself again. If preoccupied, worried and frenetic, find your way back to present reality by looking around the room at objects in turn, really seeing them as if for the first time. Listening to sounds of traffic, for example, is excellent for slowing down the mind. Just listen as if the city noises were the sounds of instruments in an orchestra and let them in without judging or evaluating them. Try to do something each day just for the pure enjoyment of it, something that has nothing at all to do with work or 'getting it together'. This could be anything from going for a walk to reading or watching television. The latter, though, has to be treated with caution, for too much television can be a strain on the eyes or leave you over-stimulated so that you might not be able to sleep afterwards. It is good to give the eyes a complete rest for maybe ten minutes every day by shutting out light completely, perhaps using a blindfold.

You may not be able to shut out noise so completely, but at least you can choose what to listen to. Listening to music is a beautiful way to unwind, as is of course playing it if you can. It is tremendously evocative of mood, and with the right sort of music you can create a very relaxing atmosphere. For this purpose instrumental music is usually better than vocal, and slow or flowing music better than fast or dance tempos. 'New Age' type music is ideal for our quieter moments and composers like Jarre, Vangelis, Halpen, Kitaro and Deuter have produced albums and tapes which are ideal for putting on when you have just got home from work, for example. Their type of music has a freshness, lightness and flowing quality which is just right when you stagger in feeling anything *but* fresh, light or flowing. Also on the market are tapes of 'environmental sounds' such as waves breaking on the surf, or the cries of seabirds. Others of fountains playing or the sounds of the countryside are also restful.

Whichever way we do it, somehow we must counteract the constant overloading of our nervous system by the massive input of stimuli around us. Allow time for unwinding, for example, after exposure to crowds, rush and noise on a shopping expedition or after battling your way home through the evening rush hour. Firmly resist the clamours for attention of those who may be waiting for you at home when you return or you will end up as harassed as poor Anne whose elderly mother makes demands on her as soon as she's inside the front door. Insist on taking your space for a while and, if that is a problem for others, explain that this is what you need to do for yourself right now so that they don't feel rejected. They may do so anyway, but that is their choice. Sometimes you won't even need to withdraw, but just let someone wait on you for a change and make the tea or the evening meal. Remember always that you have to 'switch off' before you can 'turn on' again. Unless you do, the merry-go-round gets to be merry hell!

CHAPTER FIVE

Deep Body Relaxation

This chapter deals with ways of accumulating energy, allowing it to build up again after we have been losing it – a process which happens naturally whenever we allow ourselves to be still, silent and in touch with our bodies. For most of the day we are 'out there' earning our living, relating, travelling and usually unaware of what is going on with our bodies and our body energy. This is why we overdo things and get fatigued, for we are not sufficiently aware of when to ease up. Body awareness is not only crucial to relaxation, it *is* relaxation. Whenever we are in pain, for example, we tense ourselves up, but if we can allow ourselves to really feel the pain much of this tension will disperse. We may still have the pain (or this too may disappear if it is arising from tension itself) but we shall feel more comfortable if we don't resist it with fear and irritation. Much tension and fatigue is the result of spending far too long thinking, worrying and generally living frenetically. By giving our attention to the body, energy comes back into it, for as we have suggested, our energy goes where our attention is. The experience that goes with attention-energy being centred in the body is relaxation, sensuality and, with luck, bliss – so body awareness is well worth cultivating!

Yoga

It was in India that relaxation and the intentional accumulation of vital energy ('prana') was developed into the system called hatha yoga. Unlike Western forms of exercise which develop muscles and stamina, this form of yoga relies on postures which work on the endocrine and nervous systems to promote serenity and suppleness. Over the last ten years or so, yoga has become popular in the West and books and classes are readily available. Try the postures described below to see if yoga is for you, in which case you could explore it further with a teacher. These postures should be attempted on an empty stomach, so allow 3–4 hours after a heavy meal, 2 hours after a light meal. Wear the minimum of clothing, but make sure you are warm enough. Move into and out of the postures gently and slowly and hold them only for as long as feels comfortable. Never strain. Breathing should be normal; rest for a while between postures. The names of some of these postures suggest that the first yogis got their ideas from observing Nature: the lotus, the mountain, the tree, the locust, the lion – yes, there are still lions in the Gujarat province of India.

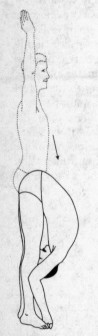

Bending Forward

Bending Forward
This pose invigorates the whole body. Keeping the feet together, inhale deeply, raise the arms above the head and then, while exhaling, bend over and grasp the big toes, ankles or calves (whichever is the furthest you can reach without bending your knees). When the exhalation is complete, bend the head down to touch the knees. Hold this position for a few seconds. Do not force. Return to a standing position, take a deep breath and repeat several more times.

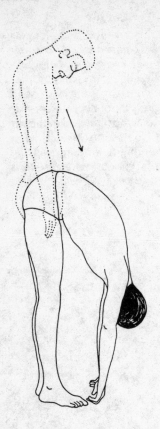

The 'Droop'

The 'Droop'

If you feel that Bending Forward was beyond the limits of your suppleness, try this variation which is less invigorating but more relaxing. Stand with the feet slightly apart, arms hanging down by the sides. Let your chin drop and the shoulders sag. Very, very slowly continue this downward-bending movement. Keep the legs straight, look at your feet and allow the head to float gently down towards them as far as it will go. Your arms will now be hanging down in front of you with the hands open. Try, without straining, to touch your toes. Hold this position for a few moments and then, as slowly as you went down, start to uncoil until you finish in an upright position, arms at the sides. Breathe out as you go down, inhale as you come up.

The Tree

Stand with the feet shoulder-width apart. Bring up the left foot and place the heel in the right groin (or as close as you can get). DON'T break your leg by trying too hard! Keeping the foot there, clasp the hands behind the neck, straighten the back and gaze at a point ahead of you and slightly above eye-level. You will probably wobble at first, so it might be safer to stand close to a wall so that you can use it to help keep your balance. Breathe normally and

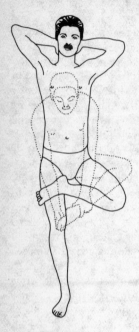

hold this posture for as long as feels comfortable without straining. To come out of it, use your hands to free the left foot from the right groin and stand straight again. Repeat, but this time with the right heel in the left groin. This posture is really good for calming down and centring again whenever you feel restless or disturbed.

The Tree

The Folded Leaf

From being a tree, become a 'folded leaf'. Get down on your knees and assume an umbilical position, forearms and forehead on the floor, hands gently clasping your head. Keep the buttocks low and relax as long as you want in this comfortable and reassuring foetal posture.

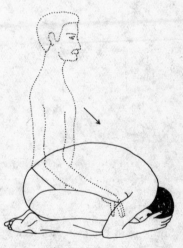

The Folded Leaf

The Cobra

From the Folded Leaf, move straight into the Cobra. Uncoil your length and raise the upper part of the body, supporting it on elbows and forearms, hands flat on the floor in front of you. Belly, thighs and knees remain in contact with the floor throughout this posture, as do the insteps. Pressing on hands and forearms, raise the torso as high as is comfortable – and then a little more. While in this position raise the chin, open the mouth and let the tongue protrude as much as possible. Hold, relax and flex forearms slowly to bring you down to a prone position full-length on the floor. After resting for a few moments, repeat the raising of the torso, mouth open, tongue protruding. Hold, then down again. This posture is particularly good for stretching the spine and relaxing the face and is also invigorating.

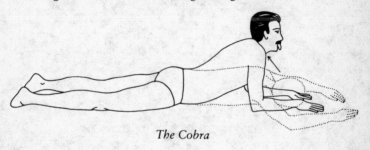

The Cobra

Reversed Corpse

From the Cobra, stretch out so that you are lying face down full-length on the floor, just as you do when sunbathing and trying to get your back tanned. Arms can be stretched out ahead of you or at the sides, whichever is more comfortable. Take a few deep breaths. Relax, feel your body getting heavier and the floor supporting its weight.

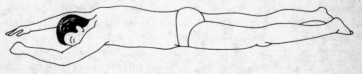

Reversed Corpse

Prarthana

A variation of the Reversed Corpse, this is even more relaxing, as much for the feelings as for the body. Prarthana has long been used as a posture for meditation and prayer. Stay lying on your stomach full-length. Place one instep (either will do) over the other sole. Place the fingers of one hand over the fingers of the other and rest your forehead on the upper hand so that the latter presses on the 'third eye' between the eyebrows. Rest in this position for as long as you want.

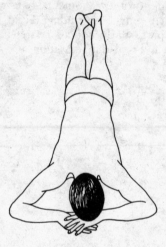

Prathna

Shoulderstand

(Do not attempt this posture if you suffer from chest complaints or high blood pressure. Rest immediately if you feel dizzy or get spots before the eyes.) Roll over on to your back, arms at the sides. Slowly draw both knees up and, using your elbows, forearms and hands as levers, *gently* roll up into an inverted position, supporting your weight on the shoulders. Legs should be straight up with the toes pointing at the ceiling or at the top of the wall behind your head. Hands should now shift so as to hold the lower back to help stop you rolling back down again. Stay like this in the inverted position for a few seconds only and relax into it. Then come down slowly and rest in the Basic Relaxed Posture (described below) for at least five minutes. The Shoulderstand relaxes the legs – it's good for varicose veins and excellent after being on your feet all day – reverses the pull of gravity on the internal organs, and refreshes the lungs, face and brain with increased blood circulation.

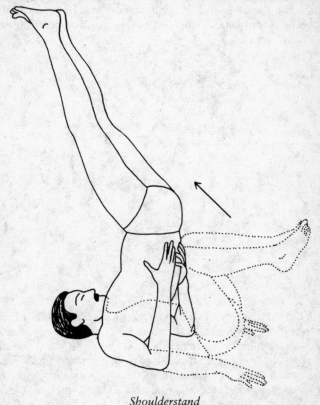

Shoulderstand

The Lion
One of the things that practising yoga postures does for you is to make you look fresher and younger, quite apart from relaxing you and giving you more energy. The Lion is a good one to do when

you catch yourself in the mirror and wince at seeing how washed-out you look! It will also help to clear up sore throats or bring back the voice you've 'lost' from talking too much. Sit on your heels and place your hands on the knees. Take a deep breath, exhale and stick out your tongue as far as it goes without gagging. Open up the mouth and eyes, stiffen the fingers and spread them apart. Tense the neck and throat and the whole body. Hold the position for a few seconds, then relax. Repeat from the beginning two or three times.

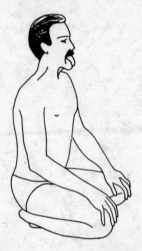

Trying out these postures will give you some idea of the power of yoga to ease tension, refresh and restore energy and to rejuvenate. They have been practised for at least six thousand years and the early yogis deserve our gratitude for passing on their first-hand experience of what helped them to relax – basically, restoring body awareness in stillness and silence. The 'Father of Yoga', Patanjali, was the first to actually set things down in writing in the fourth century BC in the Yoga Sutras. Before that the techniques, which also include breathing exercises (pranayama) and dieting, were handed down verbally from master to disciple.

As well as using the formal postures of yoga, we can invent our own. Try out your own ways of making your body feel more relaxed by tuning in to what it wants to do next. Anything that *feels* right *is* right when it comes to easing tension, for your body knows best what it needs to feel good again. Experiment, for example, with stretching, squatting, rolling the shoulders, shaking the whole body, exercising the neck – even crawling around on all fours like a cat. Incidentally, there is a lot to be learned from observing cats, the most relaxed and graceful of creatures (quite apart from the relaxing effect of fondling and stroking one). Be a cat, for example, when you wake up and before you get out of bed in the morning. Stretch, yawn, push down each leg in turn as if trying to make it longer. To leap out of bed straightaway is to 'get out of bed the wrong way' – a jarring start to the day that will not leave you feeling much like purring. Learn too from the cat how economical it is with its energy: its ability to be intensely concentrated on stalking a bird one moment, and when the bird flies away, just sitting – a real meditator!

Sessions of yoga should always end with the basic relaxation exercise now to be described in some detail because it is the simplest, fastest way of accumulating energy and of relaxing totally. It is in fact a hatha yoga posture with the unfortunate name of 'The Corpse' – just right for when you come home dead beat, dying to relax!

Basic Relaxation Exercise
Make sure that you will not be disturbed for at least half an hour; also that the room is warm enough. Loosen clothing and take off your shoes. Turn down the lighting so that the room is dimly lit. Lie down either on a firm mattress or on a carpeted floor with the head either unsupported or resting on a low pillow. Put on a blindfold. Arms should be at the sides, palms up or down whichever feels more relaxed. Take a few deep, slow breaths and start silently repeating the word 'Relax' as you exhale. Have the intention to set aside for a while any problems with which you may have been preoccupied (yes, including THAT one) and tell yourself that you will deal with them later.

Listen to the sounds from the outside world that come to you as you lie there with your eyes closed, without trying to identify them or wishing they were not there. Feel your body getting heavier and heavier and allow the mattress or the floor to take on the responsibility for supporting your weight. As you feel yourself sinking into the floor, let your mouth drop open and the muscles of your face sag. Give yourself permission to really *feel* how tired you are and to let this show in your expression. Become aware of your breathing, through the mouth from now on. Sigh deeply a few times, then continue breathing normally (but through the mouth).

Start now to bring energy down from the head into the body by giving attention to the various parts in turn. Try to really *feel* them, knowing that by doing so you are energizing them. Begin with the toes of the left foot; don't wriggle them – just feel them 'from the inside', one toe after the other. Now feel the rest of the left foot in turn: the heel pressing into the floor or mattress, the sensitive sole, the hard bones on the top of the instep . . . Give yourself as much time as you need, for this is also an exercise in slowing down. Now feel the weight of the whole foot, imagining it getting heavier and sinking into the floor.

Next, move on to the left ankle. Feel its shape and the hard protuberances each side of it. After lingering a while, move on upwards. Feel the length of the shinbone and its hardness. Tense up the muscle of the calf and then relax it, feeling its softness expanding out on to the floor. Tighten the muscle again and relax it again. Feel the left calf getting heavier and let it do so, trusting the floor to support it. Go on up to the left knee-cap: its shape, size and hardness and the soft area behind it. Move your attention now up to the thigh and feel the length of the femur, the large bone inside it. Tighten up the big muscle above it – then relax it. Tighten it up again, and relax it again. Take your time . . . Now feel the *whole* left leg getting heavier and heavier, sinking down . . . feel the difference between this leg and the unrelaxed right leg. After a few moments, starting with the toes of the right foot, go through the same process with the other leg.

Enjoy the blissful sensation of heaviness in your limbs which will start spreading throughout the rest of your body even before you begin working on the other parts. The technique is the same all over: if it is a muscle, first tighten it then relax it, tighten it again, relax it again – and allow it to get heavier. Otherwise, feel the part as much as you can, its shape, size and texture. The constant theme, whichever part it is, should be 'heaviness, letting-go, sinking down'.

When the legs are totally relaxed, continue with the following sequence:

buttocks
anus (tighten/relax)
genitals (tighten/relax)
lower back
spine
shoulders
left arm (upper, elbow, forearm, wrist)
left hand (palm, back, thumb, fingers)
right arm (upper, elbow, forearm, wrist)
right hand (palm, back, thumb, fingers)
belly (spend a lot of time on the belly, for it is likely to be tight. The feeling you want to end up with here is 'soft-bellied', wide open with 'guts' exposed. Don't force, rather *allow* this opening-up to happen.)
chest (breathe slow and deep, like sighing, into the heart area and feel that you are cleansing and energizing the heart.)

Feel the whole weight of your torso on the floor getting heavier and heavier. Enjoy this delicious sensation before moving on to the head. Feel the back of your head pressing into the floor, supported by it as you allow it to get heavier. Feel the scalp and the hair follicles (how many are there?) Feel where there is tension in the face; make it more tense by screwing it up – and relaxing it. Screw up the face again as tightly as you can, frown, clench the teeth – then relax, letting your chin drop with a deep sigh. Allow yourself to look as exhausted, discouraged or 'untogether' as you may have been feeling during the day and exaggerate this with your facial expression.

By now, however, you should be as blissfully relaxed as you have ever been in your life. Just enjoy it for as long as you feel able to (and be generous with yourself for a change!), letting your body get heavier and heavier. Whatever comes in the way of body sensations, feelings or thoughts, just allow to be there. Experience them, let them come and let them go . . . Be totally passive, just a witness, an experiencer, as if you were meditating. And remember, if any thought is particularly disturbing or charged with energy, you know how to handle it: give attention to your breathing, to the hara and to sounds from the outside. The state of deep relaxation that you are in is like being asleep except that a part of you remains awake. Unless, of course, you 'drop off', in which case you will feel as refreshed when you come to after a short while as if you had had several hours' sleep. The Basic Relaxation Exercise is an excellent thing to do on those nights when you get to bed and find that you are so wound up you can't sleep – and, as we shall see later when we consider how to handle insomnia, a 'must' for insomniacs. The exercise is also a marvellous way to recharge your batteries after work if you are planning to go out 'on the town' or to a social engagement and don't really have time to take a nap beforehand. It might be a good idea to set the alarm however, just in case you do fall into a deep sleep and ruin everything by having to rush again to get ready to go out!

The Exercise is so effective because it kills so many birds with one stone. While you are doing it you are slowing down, practising body awareness, taking your space and keeping energy well and truly 'in'. While listening to outer sounds you practise present-centredness, that is, staying in touch with what is really going on right now in and around you, centred in your body rather than in thoughts of past and future inside your head. Wearing the blindfold, sense withdrawal stops you losing energy. You might want to shut out sounds as well as by using earplugs, but I have yet to find any that do more than merely *muffle* noise. Unless you are really thirsty for silence (or the closest one ever gets to it these days) the Exercise could be enhanced by playing (softly, of course) an apropriately restful piece of background music. The 'New Age' tapes are very good for this with their synthesizers and general spaciness, while best of all might be the environmental 'Ocean' tape of waves crashing on to the beach (see Appendix). The latter is particularly effective if you choose to do a visualization in the last stage of the Basic Relaxation Exercise (i.e. when you have finished creating total body awareness and are just relaxing into it).

Visualizations

Visualizations can be a beautifully effective way to promote relaxation as well as a real treat. To visualize something is simply to create an image or scene in your mind and to dwell upon it. We do it all the time when we daydream or fantasize about, say, winning the pools – which may make us feel less uptight about the bills that have just come through the letter-box or that letter from the bank manager. We all know that we can be moved to tears when watching a real 'weepie' or return home paranoid enough to turn on all the lights in the house and inspect every room after being shaken up by a 'creepie' – even though we know quite well that 'it was only a film'. Visualizations are our own 'home movies' which, like real movies, have the power not only to stir up feelings within us but also to affect physiological reactions. The body will prepare itself for the business of fight or flight in the same way whether the threat is real or only imagined to be real. A few years ago while I was living in India, I came down into the kitchen during the night to get a drink as it was stiflingly hot, just before the monsoon. Opening the door I switched on the light – and stepped on what looked and felt like a large, coiled-up snake. To say that adrenalin flowed would be a gross understatement – my shriek of sheer panic as I nearly hit the ceiling aroused the whole house. Even when the source of my fright was identified as merely a thick piece of old rope left behind by the Indian workers we had had in that day, it took some minutes before my heart-rate and respiration returned to normal – and *much* longer before I was able to see the funny side of it.

In the kitchens of our minds we cook up our own version of what is sometimes making not only snakes out of old rope, but mountains out of molehills. We shall be discussing in a later chapter how to reverse this process so as to handle emotional tension by using positive visualizations. But their effectiveness in helping the body relax and even heal itself is proven too. The work of the Simontons at Fort Worth, Texas has shown that even cancer can sometimes be responsive to deliberate positive visual-izations by patients, facilitated by the doctor treating them. Dr Carl Simonton's first patient, for example, visualized healthy cells attacking and defeating cancer cells and the amelioration in his condition was immediate and striking. Subsequently comparing the progress of patients on visualization therapy with those who were not, Simonton found that the survival period for the visualizers was about twice as long as that for the nonvisualizers and, occasionally, their cancers ceased to spread and they were able to return to normal life. In Britain too, orthodox treatment of cancer is beginning to realize the importance of the mind's role, notably at the Bristol Cancer Help Centre. It is therefore not surprising that visualizations can help to disperse our much more innocent fatigue and tension. Here are a few to give you the hang of it – and then you're on your own to enjoy yourself as you wish!

Visualization 1: Beach

This visualization obviously would go very well with the 'Ocean' tape. All visualizations should be done lying in the Basic Relaxation Posture.

Imagine the most inviting beach you can think of, perhaps one that you know already and have enjoyed. See in your mind's eye all the features of the beach scene that make it so inviting for you. Is it the ocean – vast, green, cool, flecked perhaps with white or tremendously calm? Can you see sails in the distance, or is it clear right out to the horizon? See the colour of the sand, perhaps with large rocks here and there and maybe fringed with palm trees or flowering shrubs. Feel yourself there, part of that scene. What are you doing? Swimming perhaps, or floating on your back, eyes closed in the bright sunshine warming your face while the seabirds wheel and cry overhead in the bluest of skies. Perhaps you are not swimming at all, but lying in the surf, letting the waves break and swirl over and around you, enjoying the ebb and flow, the coolness of the water on your body. See yourself later relaxing full-length on your towel, luxuriating in the warmth of the sun, feeling all the tension in your body dispersing with the drops of water evaporating on it. Are you alone or are you with a good companion? If the latter, turn over and enjoy the experience of having your back and legs massaged gently with suntan oil. Smell the fragrance of the oil and enjoy surrendering to the caring attention of this person whom you trust and with whom you feel totally at ease. Relax, enjoy and let your visualization take it from there . . .

Visualization 2: Happy Times
Cast your mind back to a time in your life when you did not have a care in the world and were very happy. Keep focusing on that contented period until a particular episode or scene begins to emerge. Recreate that event or scene in as much detail as possible. Where exactly was it, who was there, what (if anything) was said? What exactly were your feelings at this time? Re-experience them as fully as you can.

Visualization 3: Garden
Let your mind's eye roam through some of the gardens you have been in. See a succession of brilliantly-coloured flowers, beautifully trimmed lawns, trees and shrubs. Is there one special garden where you have relaxed in the past, enjoying its solitude, peace and fragrance? If no particular garden wants to be enjoyed right now, create your own ideal one. Spare no expense. You can have anything you choose in your garden, including fountains, avenues of azaleas and rhododendrons, peacocks strutting on the well-kept lawns . . . The sun of course will be shining all the time and you will be either basking in its warmth or perhaps sitting in the shade by the fish-pond, watching the gold shapes swimming lazily in and out of the water-lilies. Listen to the sounds in your garden: sweet, insistent bird song, the gentle splashing of the fountain, perhaps the buzzing of crickets invisible and tireless, the distant drone of a plane just visible high above, leaving a snow-white trail in the blue summer sky . . .

Some people have difficulty in thinking in images, in visualizing. No matter. The relaxation comes not from the visualization itself, but from its evocative effect on the feelings. If the actual pictures will not come, it will be just as effectve to *feel* what it would be like to be lying on a beach in the sun, lazing in a beautiful garden on a hot summer afternoon, being in a situation where you feel totally secure, loved and supported . . . Enjoy the blissful fantasy for as long as you have time, and make sure you also allow time for 'coming round' afterwards. It can be jarring to come straight off a beach paradise or from Eden into the noisy asphalt and concrete reality of urban living – especially if it's raining! At the end of a visualization, ground yourself again in the following way: open your eyes, stretch your body, look around the room taking in the familiar furniture and objects one by one. When you get up, do so gently. Try to keep the feelings of relaxation in your body for as long as possible by taking things as easy as you can for as long as you can.

Autogenics

Visualization is one of the techniques used in autogenics, which is about *choosing* to relax and feeling how *you* want to feel, rather than waiting for someone or something to do it for you. Brought from Canada to Britain by Dr Malcolm Carruthers in the 1970s, autogenics consists of mental exercises aimed at switching off the body's responses to stress and activating its relaxation response instead. These techniques involve taking responsibility for your own tension and fatigue and dispersing it by simple awareness exercises that transform the body's energy. When these exercises have been mastered and confidence has been gained, the *feel* of blissful, deep relaxation (or of positive mental states, whichever you are after) can be recalled at will. This is done by simply remembering the sensations and perhaps repeating a word or phrase that describes them or is associated with the experience. Next time you do the Basic Relaxation Exercise and reach a state of total body relaxation, try to pin a label on exactly how it feels to be so blissfully relaxed (itself a possible label). When you have pinpointed how total body relaxation feels for you, use the word or phrase as a mantra to repeat to yourself whenever you feel that things are getting on top of you. It will make you feel better, slow you down and tide you over until the next opportunity comes to sink totally into relaxing once more.

That these autogenic techniques really do have a powerful effect on the body as well as changing our mental states has been demonstrated objectively in biofeedback, where the physiological responses of subjects have been monitored on sensitive machines which record changes in heart-rate, blood pressure, skin con-ductivity and respiration. The power of the mind to virtually suspend even essential bodily functions is indicated in the spectacular and somewhat scary things advanced yogis can achieve. One such yogi, a man named Haridas, apparently had himself buried alive in 1837 for forty days in Lahore (in what is now Pakistan). This feat was solemnly attested to by witnesses of such impeccable credentials as the British Consul and the local military commander, a Colonel Sir Claude Wade. The spoon-bending powers of Uri Geller in more recent times not only baffled television audiences but apparently caused some consternation outside the studio too, when cutlery in households all over the country started to go haywire. Experiments have been carried out – backed up by photographs – on the effect of dispersing cloud formations simply by willing them to do so; though of course the cloud might have been doing its own thing anyway! Nevertheless, the ability to change the weather by concentrated thought is a power sometimes attributed by disciples to their gurus, for example Bubba Free John in America. In his ashram in India too, Sai Baba's casual manifestation of 'vibuti' (a fine grey powder), apparently out of thin air, is one of the party tricks he performs regularly before the astonished eyes of vast crowds.

Auto-suggestion

Fortunately most of us do not possess these strange and controversial powers to bend matter to our will and probably would not want to do so anyway. But do not underestimate your power over *yourself*: to *choose* to feel the way you would *like* to feel. Remember that nobody is born a victim, but we can end up feeling like victims when we make the wrong choices or allow things to happen that do not nourish us, either because we are unaware or just not clear or strong enough to say 'No'. We create our own fatigue by not being discriminating – about commitments, time, space, eating properly, about our needs, what we look at, listen to and surround ourselves with. Our fatigue is our responsibility too, not only because we created it but because nobody else can beat it but us. As has already been said, we are on our own. But the other side of the coin of responsibility is power and, using autogenics, we use the power of thought to change feelings and the power of feelings to mobilize energy in the body. If any reader doubts this power exists, think how easy it is to work yourself up into a rage by brooding over some imagined (or real) injustice: before you know it your jaw is tight, fists are clenched and you are ready to give battle. Alternatively, remember how tense worrying makes you feel, as with furrowed brow you pace restlessly up and down.

Just as we can use this power to make ourselves angry, nostalgic or depressed, so too we can utilize it to induce relaxation and euphoria. Auto-suggestion is most effective when the mind is not very active and other thoughts are not there to compete with our own suggestions that we relax. We are most susceptible to what amounts to self-hypnosis, therefore, at the following times: just before falling asleep; immediately upon waking; in the last stage of the Basic Relaxation Exercise; after a preliminary slowing down of the mind.

In a later chapter we shall be dealing with the uses of auto-suggestion in handling emotional tension, in which case it would be more appropriate to practise it as a preparation for a busy day out in the world, or to soothe the knocks received in the course of this. For the purpose of helping to relax, auto-suggestion is effective always during the periods set aside for unwinding and, when we are used to it, at any other time of the day whenever we feel frenetic or uptight.

Whether you do it lying in the Basic Relaxation Posture or sitting comfortably in a chair, first of all get yourself into that limbo between waking and sleeping by slow, regular breathing, sense withdrawal, body awareness and giving attention in particular to the hara. Some hypnotists suggest counting, usually backwards either from one hundred, or from ten (and if necessary starting again at 'ten'). You are ready to begin auto-suggestion when you feel drowsy, relaxed, totally in your body, aware of little else but body sensations and occasional sounds from the outside. Your subconscious now will be wide open to suggestions, so make sure you programme it properly. Once a seed is sown it will germinate sooner or later and, if it is unwelcome, it will be as tricky to eradicate as a weed. You can programme your mind-computer for the present or for the future. Here are some of the key ideas you might like to try.

PRESENT PROGRAMMING
'I am feeling more and more relaxed and blissful every moment.'
(Repeat silently several times, feeling and *believing* the words. Go
deeper and deeper into body-awareness and, after a while,
abbreviate to simply 'More and more relaxed . . . blissful . . .
relaxed . . . bliss . . .' 'Now I'm letting-go of *everything* . . .
sinking down . . . letting-go . . . down . . .' 'I feel so good . . . so
peaceful inside . . . so good . . . peace . . . peaceful.'

These, after you get the hang of them and feel their effect, can be
used like mantras at any time during a busy day, sitting on the
tube in the rush hour or whenever the crowds are getting you
down. Repeat key mantras to yourself, feel them in your hara
region while unfocusing your eyes to keep energy in and avoid
losing it.

FUTURE PROGRAMMING
We are programming ourselves all the time without being aware
that we are doing so. More often than not these programmes are
negative and, rather like prophecies, self-fulfilling. What are
prejudices after all but negative expectations? Perception, it has
been established by psychologists, is selective: we tend to
experience only what we expect to experience, to see only what
we have been conditioned to see. For example, if we get dragged
off to a dinner-party in the expectation that it will be a dreary
affair, very probably it will turn out to be so: we shall not only be
bored but boring. Unless, of course, we have decided to make the
best of it – in other words, a new intention has cancelled out the
negative expectation – in which case it may not. Intention is all-
important in pre-setting expectations and mobilizing energy, for
as has been suggested, energy follows intention. Therefore if,
before leaving the house in the morning, you form the deliberate
intention to have a good day *whatever happens*, you are pretty
sure to do so. How exactly it works is mysterious: whether
positive energy attracts positive experiences like a magnet,
whether the mind is pre-set to enjoy and not looking for trouble or
something to complain about . . . but work it does. Programme
yourself not to be so het-up or irritable – or whatever you feel has
been draining you – by using these forumulae:

'From now on I'm taking things easier . . . slow down . . . easier . . . slower . . .' (Suggestions should not only be positive of course. They should also be phrased in the positive form: not, for example, 'I'm not going to rush etc.')

'Everything will flow so smoothly at work tomorrow . . . smooth . . . flowing . . .'

'I'm going to feel full of energy this evening and have a really good time . . . full of energy . . . happy . . . happy . . . fun . . . high energy . . .'

'Every day, in every way, my life will be more and more relaxed and easy . . . more relaxed . . . easy . . . more relaxed, more relaxed . . . easier and easier . . .'

'From now on I'm looking after myself better . . . taking my time . . . more space . . . being good to myself . . . taking my time . . . looking after myself . . .'

Once again, really *feel* what you are saying and speak as if you were delivering the Ten Commandments. The more deliberate you are, the more certainty and authority you bring to your words and the more quickly they will manifest in your experience. For we act on what we believe to be true.

Bathing

The deeper you go into body awareness, the more blissful you feel. As we have seen, one of the quickest ways to get the energy out of your head – thinking, worrying and so on – is to listen to outside sounds, to take in the room with your eyes, to stretch, breathe deeply and to open up the body posture. To 'lose your mind' in fact, you have to 'come to your senses'. Sensuality relaxes the body. Witness again the cat, rubbing up against its owner's leg, tail erect, purring away; or lying on its back having its tummy tickled, legs in the air, eyes glazing over with the sheer pleasure of it all.

Bathing has long been one of mankind's favourite ways of relaxing into the body and making it feel good. Whether it is in the sea, under a shower or in a jacuzzi, we emerge feeling refreshed and cleansed at some level deeper than merely having washed sweat off our bodies, for water purifies our whole energy field as well. The ancient world revelled in bathtime to the point of decadence. Whether Cleopatra or Roman matrons ever actually bathed in asses' milk, we shall never know. But the huge ruins of the public Roman baths are evidence today of the importance they attributed to bathing as a way to relax. In the heyday of the Roman Empire people came from all over Europe to Aquae Sulis (now modern Bath) to enjoy its palatial buildings and sophisticated facilities. In that vast complex of heated rooms and pools they would sweat it out, have their bodies scraped clean with the strygil, bathe, be oiled and massaged. They would spend the best part of their day there, doing business and gossiping, perhaps nibbling honey-cakes and sipping wine, but above all relaxing and having a good time. With its gymnasia and its opportunities for social contact, Bath was the Roman equivalent of a combined modern health club and pub.

Except for the diminishing number of people who don't have bathrooms at home, public baths today are intended mainly for relaxation. The sauna has overtaken the Turkish bath in popularity these days and can be found in most towns. Many of course are 'clip-joints,' but the respectable establishments provide an ideal way of unwinding after work or on a day off. It could be a good investment for your health and the quality of your life to join a health club, if only because being a paid-up member will probably be an incentive to get your money's worth and therefore be a means of structuring space for relaxation after your working day. The more imaginative establishments do all the right things to help their clients unwind: subdued lighting, soft music, the sound of running water or a splashing jacuzzi, lots of plants, perhaps a pool with goldfish or an aquarium, quiet rooms to doze off in or to watch TV over tea and toast (or, if slimming, a juice).

Nobody would want to take a sauna every day: not only would this be expensive, it would not be advisable since it could be depleting if done too often and especially so for anyone with a weak heart. But we can take a bath every day and transform the humble bath-time at home into a deliciously sensual experience to relax our bodies. Think for a moment, what makes taking a bath relaxing at all? Firstly, is it not the *privacy*, knowing that at least for a while you can really be alone with yourself and your thoughts? The bathroom is one of the few places left in the world where one's right to privacy is still respected. 'Sorry, I was in the bath', effectively silences any complaints that you were not available when somebody phoned, called or otherwise wanted you. Secondly, there is something intrinsically relaxing in taking off one's clothes and being naked (in appropriate conditions of course, otherwise it could be quite the reverse of relaxing!). This is the appeal of naturism and of nude bathing, to which the authorities in an increasing number of holiday resorts are extending a more tolerant policy. It is not only enjoyment of the feel of the sun and air on the whole body, but also the sense of freedom and childlike innocence you get when running into the sea in your birthday suit, playing, splashing, body-surfing . . . It is a relief to strip off along with our clothes the social roles and responsibilities that go with them. Thirdly, warmth relaxes the body too, whether it is the warmth of the sun or bath water. We expand and loosen up with the heat, while cold and tension serve to contract us.

So make the most of the daily bath or shower, take your time over it and turn it into a deliciously sensual experience rather than a mere cleaning ritual. Set the scene while the bath is running. Put on some music you really like and find relaxing, perhaps light a candle or nightlight and switch off the main light. Bathing by candlelight makes the whole thing more of a treat, less functional. So does wallowing in bath water perfumed with oil of your favourite fragrance. Quite apart from the aesthetics, according to aromatherapists certain fragrances have special relaxing properties – among them lavender, sandalwood, rose and cedarwood. Don't have the water too hot and don't stay in too long, otherwise you may feel enervated afterwards. But soak and enjoy, unwind and drowse, allowing the tension accumulated during the day to melt away together with the grime and sweat. Washing the hair is relaxing too, for it disperses the energy that clings to the hair after too much worrying or concentrating. Often, if taking a bath is out of the question because it is the wrong time or place, just soaking the hands up to the wrists in water as hot as you can bear will have a soothing effect.

Massage

After bathing, lie on your bed for a while in the Basic Relaxation

Posture. It will probably not be necessary to do the exercise to get into body awareness, since you will almost certainly be there already. An excellent tape to play at this stage would be the environmental one of the sound of ocean waves. This is also the very best time to be massaged, either by a friend or visiting professional – or if in a sauna of course, by the resident masseur/masseuse.

As well as helping us to relax and being a pleasurable and sensual experience, massage heightens vitality, tones muscles, removes toxins and stimulates the circulation. It is therefore a good thing to have on a regular basis, especially if you live a hectic life and can afford the money but don't have much time. Make sure, however, that you get a massage that will leave you relaxed and not shaken up by being hacked, slapped and generally pulled about. It helps the person giving you the massage if you tell them how you are feeling, where you have any aches and feelings of tension, and any particular parts of the body to which you would like them to give special attention – the feet, perhaps, or the lower back or shoulders. Make it clear to them whether you want a relaxing massage (Esalen or sensual massage) or a stimulating, energizing one (Swedish or shiatsu). While being massaged, surrender more and more to the ministrations of the soothing hands working to relax your body. Just let go, give up trying to control everything for a change and trust the other person totally. Let your attention follow the sensations that arise as you are stroked, kneaded and so on: relax into them, let your body get heavier and heavier – and enjoy it.

Self-massage

Sometimes after a bath you may feel like a massage, but there is nobody around to give you one. In this case, try giving yourself a massage. This is not as strange as it may sound for we do it all the time, albeit unconsciously. Think, for example, how we rub a bump or a bruise, scratch our heads when puzzled, rub our hands in satisfaction or wring them in despair. Nor is self-massage as difficult as one might imagine if the simple routine described below is followed. Quite apart from the purely physical benefits, there are certain psychological advantages from giving caring awareness and attention to one's own body. Many people have negative feelings about their bodies: they consider themselves too fat, too skinny, too this, too that – and generally not measuring up to the stereotypes currently in vogue and presented to us by the media as the only type of body worth having. Massaging your body is validating it as worthy of loving attention and, as we have seen, attention means giving it energy.

Hand massage
Starting with the hands will energize the hands themselves, ready for massaging.

Rub hard with the thumb of one hand from the side of the other hand (furthest away from the thumb) into the centre of the palm, several times. Pinch the fleshy part of the palm next to the thumb a

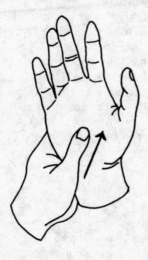

few times. Pull each thumb and finger with a corkscrew motion (just as if you were 'cracking your knuckles'). Pinch and rub the skin between each finger. With the left thumb, massage the palm

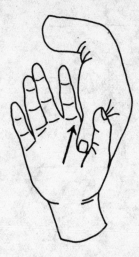

of the right hand, simultaneously massaging the back of the right hand with the rest of the left hand. Massage the left hand in the same way, using the right hand.

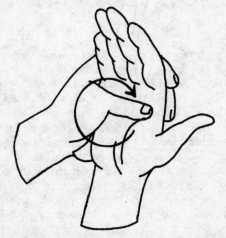

Let the hands grasp each other and squeeze together in a 'cupping' motion. Press the fingers and thumb hard against each other.

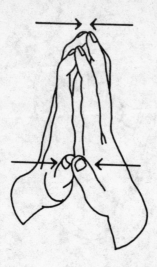

Relax them, press hard again, relax again. This is a popular technique for relaxation in Japan. Finish the hand massage by rubbing the hands together vigorously until they are quite hot.

Head massage

Bring the energy generated from rubbing the hands together to refresh the face, covering it with both hands. Take away the hands, warm them again by rubbing them together and place them over the face once more. Do this as often as feels good to you. You can, if you prefer, get the same soothing effect from using hot flannels. Have one flannel soaking, ready to use, and one covering the face. Don't scald yourself: test for heat first on the back of the hand before applying a flannel to the face. Rinse the face with cold water afterwards as an astringent and, if you like, smooth in some moisturising cream.

Smooth the forehead, from the 'frown lines' outwards to the hairline. Press firmly with the middle fingers, using both hands simultaneously. Using the third fingers, trace firmly the line of the eyebrow from the 'third eye' outwards.

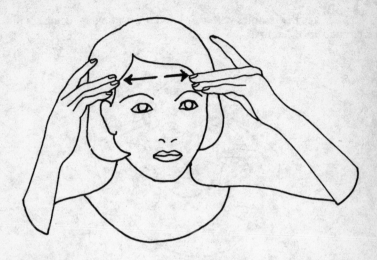

Make fists and, allowing the jaws to sag, massage them using the fists in a rocking motion, knuckles pressed into the hollows below the cheek bones. Don't break your jaw!

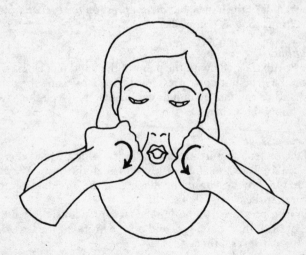

Massage the temples with third and fourth fingers, using small circular movements.

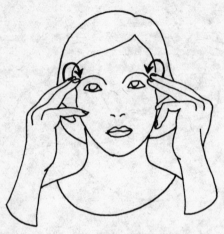

Untighten the scalp muscles by wiggling your ears (if you can), then gently apply friction and light tapping to the scalp itself, using the tips of the fingers and thumbs.

Finish the head massage by palming the eyes: cover the eyes with the palms of the hands, but *do not press on the eyeballs*. Stay like this for as long as you wish.

Belly rubbing

Just that! Rub the belly with the palm of the hand in a clockwise direction. Be firm, but don't press hard. Finish by using the palm of one hand to rub fast up and down the area between the navel and the pubis. This energizes the hara.

Meridian massage

Meridians in acupuncture are the pathways along which energy (called 'chi' in Taoist medicine) flows through the body. We can stimulate this flow of vitality by massaging the meridians in the direction that the energy flows.

Using firm pressure, run both hands simultaneously down the outside of both thighs and legs and up the inside of the legs and thighs. Repeat several times.

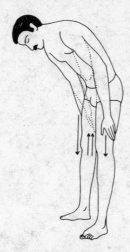

   Starting from the back of the left hand and fingers, run the right palm up the back of the left arm and down the inside of the left arm. Finish the stroke with a flick of the right hand off the fingers of the left hand. Repeat several times. Change over and work with the left hand on the right arm.

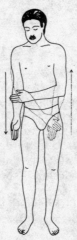

Neck massage
This is something you can do during the working day when, for example, you have been sitting too long at the typewriter or the boss is being a 'pain in the neck'!

Knead the back of the neck between the palm and fingers of both hands. Rotate the head gently, not clockwise and anti-clockwise, but up and down and left and right.

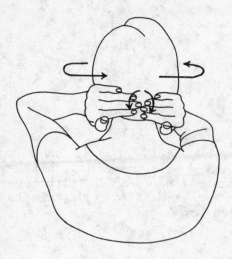

Foot massage
This too can be done whenever it would be permissible to take your shoes off and is 'de rigueur' to refresh aching feet after the rigours of being on them for too long.

First get the circulation going in the feet and loosen them up by rotating them from the ankle. Flex them and wriggle the toes.

Grasp one foot with both hands, palms and thumbs on the top of the instep. Squeeze the underside of the foot all over as firmly as you can with the fingers.

Squeeze the top of the foot with both palms, moving outwards and upwards towards the big and little toes.

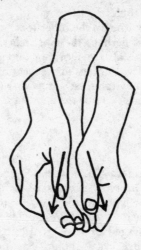

Make a fist and screw it hard into the ball of the foot and then under the arch of the instep.

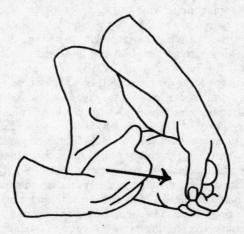

Rotate the big toe between the thumb and the index finger. Stroke and press the rest of the foot in any way that feels good. Pinch the skin between each toe in turn. This is particularly pleasurable for most people.

Repeat the whole routine on the other foot.

Massaging the feet is perhaps the most relaxing piece of self-massage you can do. It is also invigorating and grounding, while manipulation of the nerve-endings in the feet (and hands) is used in reflexology to tone up vital organs and other parts of the body with which they connect.

Exchanging Massage

One of the most relaxing ways to be with somebody you like is to exchange massages. The type of massage given will of course depend on how intimate you are and how comfortable you both feel with bodily contact. If you have already experienced the pleasure of being massaged or have tried out the self-massage routine described above, you should have no difficulty in massaging another. So long as you remain sensitive and gentle, you can't go far wrong; if you do, no doubt the recipient of your ministrations will soon let you know.

Try to stay in touch with the other person at an energy level by endeavouring to sense what they are feeling when you do a certain stroke and which parts of their body are tense and need attention next. Trust your intuition and let your hands do the rest. Remember that the aim of your massage is not deep muscle manipulation, but relaxation and the creation of a soothing and caring vibration between you. Make sure you keep a blanket near, to cover any parts of the body which are not actually being massaged and start to feel cold. It is best to be massaged on an empty stomach – and remember not to massage over fresh scar tissue or distended veins. Make the whole session a real treat for the senses with attention to lighting, fragrances and suitable soft music. It is better to bathe before rather than after a massage. If you are both going to be massaged and your intimacy is such that it is appropriate, sharing the same bath-tub beforehand can be fun, provided you don't get the tap end!

Massage on a firm but comfortable surface: use a massage table if you have one, a mattress or carpeted floor if you do not. Cover the surface with a towel first, especially if using oil. Oil makes for a pleasanter massage than if you work without it or with talcum: you can use firm strokes without tugging at body hair and causing your partner to wince and yelp. Also the fragrance of the oil adds to the sensuality of the massage. According to aromatherapists, absorbing certain oils into the skin is healing and relaxing too, and lavender and sandalwood are especially good for this.

If you are the one being worked on, all you have to do is relax and enjoy it. Should you be feeling strung up and particularly tense or frenetic, take a few deep breaths as you lie there waiting for the massage to begin, then practise the body awareness of the Basic Relaxed Posture. While being worked on, let your attention follow the sensations that arise as your friend's hands stroke, squeeze, rub or whatever. Relax into them, surrender your control, let your body become heavier, and enjoy.

If you are the one giving the massage, make sure that you have enough space to massage any part of the body from any angle: for example, that there is enough room around the mattress for you to be able to move round it. Get your friend to lie face down and start with the back. Rest your (warmed) hands on the small of the back, watch the rise and fall of your friend's breathing, and breathe in synchronicity. Stay like this for a minute or two, tuning in to your partner; when you feel ready, start massaging the back in any way that feels right. Generally we massage towards rather than away from the heart. Try also not to break contact with the body of the person being massaged too abruptly; for example, when you need to re-oil your hands, either keep one hand in contact or remove them both slowly and gently. Be very sensitive, as people open up a lot when they are being massaged. It can be jarring, for example, to be suddenly jabbed or grabbed from nowhere by cold hands, so if you have withdrawn your hands be sure to re-establish contact very gently again . . . Make sure of course that your finger-nails are short enough before you even lay a finger on anyone else.

It is good to start with the back, so that your partner does not feel too exposed too soon, and allow plenty of time, for there is usually a lot of tension there. Work on the shoulders as well, then a little more on the back before moving down to the buttocks and then to the legs; if necessary, cover the back with the blanket while you work on these. After the legs have been done, ask your friend to turn over and then massage the feet in turn. Include each toe and the spaces between the toes, for the latter is particularly pleasurable for most people. Be super-sensitive when working on the front of the body, for the most vulnerable areas are here – the abdomen and face particularly. Never press hard on the belly, the eyes or, incidentally, the spine. From the feet, work your way up: legs, belly (just gentle rubbing with the palm in a clockwise direction is enough here), chest, arms, hands (including each thumb and finger). By now you will be located at the side of the person being massaged; move to stand or sit behind the head and finish the session with a long, loving, gentle face massage.

It is up to you which strokes you use. For guidance, here are a few tips:

1   Use long firm strokes on back and legs, starting with both hands in the small of the back or on either side of the ankle, flowing up either side of the spine or leg to shoulders or buttocks and, in one continuous stroke, down the sides so as to finish up where you started. Repeat as often as feels right, then cover the same areas with light, fast downward brushing with the finger-tips.

2   Use squeezing, kneading and stroking for fleshy areas like feet, calves, thighs, hands, shoulders and upper arms.

3   Use your fingers and thumbs to trace the line of bones, e.g. ankle, kneecap, elbow, wrist, jaws.

What you are trying to do is to give the recipient of your massage an experience of his or her own body, to define to them its outline and volume. They should end up blissfully relaxed, half-dozing and totally centred in the body. It is always a reward for one's efforts to be finishing up with a face massage and to see the complete let-go on the face one is gently stroking, the blissful expression, the softness and open-ness. Where the two of you go from there is up to you. For relaxation, easy is right.

CHAPTER SIX

Handling Emotional Tension

One of the things that can drain us more quickly than anything else is emotional tension. Worry, negative feelings, unresolved problems and relationships, stress – all take up a lot of energy. We brood, torture ourselves with guilt and catastrophic expectations, feel resentment and rack our brains fruitlessly for a way out of situations in which we feel trapped and helpless. Tension is reflected in the body: restless, we lose energy all over the place, not least in irritable outbursts that we immediately regret; or, hopeless, we sink into a grey depression where no one can reach us. Appetite goes, together with our sense of humour and ability to relax, to play and to enjoy. Strained and pallid, we wonder whatever happened to the quality in our lives as we lie awake at night, desperate, confused, lost. Too often we resort to palliatives to ease our tension: tranquillizers, alcohol, compulsive eating, chain-smoking.

The cause of our tension could be stress from inside or from outside ourselves. Our relationship with ourselves may be fraught, arising from guilt or negative self-image, inferiority feelings and so forth. On the other hand, it may be that our relationships with significant people in our lives are not going well, either at home or at work. Perhaps it is worrying about health or money that is sapping our energy. The menopause, both female and male, is a time of loss of confidence, of emotional insecurity and professional misgivings: we may feel that promotion and performance, as well as time and looks, are passing us by. It is for many people a time of anxiety and fear, of being a has-been, alone and perhaps poor as well. Stress may erupt suddenly into our lives with illness, accident or bereavement, the greatest stressor of all.

Some of these causes of emotional tension need to be handled with awareness and willingness to change, and may even be harbingers of a new phase of personal growth, leading us, for example, out of old patterns of being and relating into new and fresh possibilities. Jung always suggested that the 'neurotics' amongst us (everybody?) were simply people resisting the advent of the new, which they could not handle simply because it was unfamiliar and threatening. Anyone who feels ashamed of emotional tension, of being 'uncool', should take comfort in the notion that they are very probably more sensitive to stress than others and therefore more sensitive generally. This means that you can go further into experiencing what life has to offer than the duller and more placid and thick-skinned of our brethren. You may have more lows, but you will also have more highs.

Emotional tension of itself, therefore, is not always entirely negative, even though it may not feel so good. Maybe it is life's way of putting pressure on us to make necessary changes in our life-style to enable more of ourselves to be expressed, and we shall be discussing this point further in the next chapter. Sometimes, however, we can see nothing positive at all in the nightmare and experience only a deep sense of loss. When bereavement occurs, for example, there is little we can do except live through the experience of it and to *really* experience it – and let time do the rest. One thing that we *can* and must do, nevertheless, whatever the source of our emotional tension, is to give attention to self-nourishment. We must look after ourselves at times of crisis as lovingly and as caringly as if we were nurturing the most important person in our lives. We have indeed to be our own best friend.

Dieting for Stress

The first line of defence when handling emotional tension, as for beating fatigue, must always be attention to diet. In chapter three, we suggested that protein or vitamin deficiency can be at the root of nervous exhaustion and that vitamin B was particularly crucial. Sometimes, merely stepping up the intake of B vitamins will alleviate 'nerves' – as for example, B6 in the case of premenstrual tension. Smokers may be deficient of B1, vegetarians of B12. If you take the whole complex to be on the safe side perhaps in the form of Brewer's yeast with added B12., you cannot go far wrong. A high-protein diet is essential when undergoing acute stress, in addition to extra B, C and E vitamins and extra calcium.

Certain other vitamin-like substances, as yet still unidentified, have a powerful capacity to protect humans against the results of stress. It has been found, for example, that rats are completely safeguarded from the effects of the administration of strychnine and other poisons when given food containing these 'anti-stress factors'. These factors are present in liver, kidneys, wheatgerm, soy flour and leafy green vegetables. Pantothenic acid, too, has been tested not only on rats but on humans and has been found to cut down dramatically the effects of stress on the body: it prevented a rise in blood sugar, destruction of protein and salt-retention, as well as causing blood cholesterol to fall. As far back as 1952, the National Research Council recommended 20 mg of pantothenic acid daily for sick people, to help counteract the stress of their illness. Modern nutritionists, Adelle Davis for example (*Let's Get Well*, Unwin Paperbacks), suggests that this is far too low and that it can be greatly increased without toxic effect. Bearing all this in mind, a 'stress diet' to be adopted whenever we are really 'going through it' should be high in protein, vitamins, calcium and foods containing the 'anti-stress factors'. The following should therefore be included:

liver
kidneys
soy products
leafy green vegetables
milk
cheese
fruit
wheatgerm
vitamin B complex (or Brewer's yeast with added B12)
vitamin C (high dose, 500 mg or 1 gm)
vitamin E (at least 100 iu)
pantothenic acid (B5)
ginseng (should only be taken over short periods by women

because it stimulates the male hormones)

It is essential for people who are depressed to be encouraged to eat, since loss of appetite is a particularly pernicious concomitant of acute depression. Where reluctance to eat is extreme, as a temporary resort proprietary 'nerve tonics' like Sanatogen and 'invalid diets' like Complan can be given, together with nourishing soups such as chicken, miso or vegetable. But eat they must.

Remember that tension *per se* is not always unproductive. Fear is intended by Nature to generate energy, either for flight from danger when threatened or for anger for defence when attacked (or to protect others from attack). Moreover, being 'keyed up' is perfectly appropriate before giving a performance in competitive examinations or sport, for example, or acting. Without this type of tension, the performance might well be mediocre. But emotional tension that does not find an outlet in creativity or catharsis is unpleasant and draining. It could also *impair* our performance – in public appearances and engagements when part of doing the job well entails at least *appearing* to be at ease, or in work demanding total concentration – and always casts a shadow over our enjoyment, if it even allows it. Human beings are not machines and sometimes, for no apparent reason, we may feel tense emotionally when we really need to be or would like to be relaxed. At these times, we can practise some of the techniques already described for inducing relaxation.

Breathing
Remember that changing the breathing pattern changes the mood. The old advice to 'count to ten' when about to flare up in anger is sound: it gives one 'breathing space', time for the breathing pattern to change – or even to start breathing again. Whenever you are upset, try breathing slowly and deeply into the hara to centre yourself again before taking any action – the latter is then much more likely to be 'right on', i.e. appropriate to the actual situation, a response rather than a reaction. This is especially useful at work when dealing with difficult customers or bad news. Remember too that any irritability or 'down' feeling may also be due to insufficient oxygenization of the blood and the brain, so if possible do your breathing exercise by an open window or out in the open air.

Taking time, taking space
Whenever you feel things starting to 'get on top of you', give yourself a break – literally. Slow down, open out the body posture, centre yourself in the body again and not in your head, open up the posture and, if possible, do the Basic Relaxation Exercise. Whatever time you can spare for your break – whether a visit to the wash-room, going for a walk or best of all, a holiday – TAKE IT!

Handling Insomnia

One of the worst things that happens to us when we are tense is that we can't sleep – and this at the very time when we need plenty of rest to recharge those batteries. Giving yourself adequate sleep is as important for beating fatigue and tension as is the right nourishment in the way of food. In fact, we can do without food for far longer than we can do without sleep. Yet knowing this is not only useless if one cannot sleep at nights; it actually makes things worse by producing anxiety that one's health will suffer. 'Try to get some sleep' is advice as silly as saying, 'Try to relax,' for sleep and relaxation only happen when you *stop* trying.

Here are some tips for those who dread yet another night spent wide- awake in the grey small hours, perhaps hating all those out there (or the one lying next to you) who are blissfully snoring their heads off.

DURING THE DAY
Make sure you get enough exercise and fresh air. If you are not working, move the body: go for a long walk, clean the house, go to dance class – anything that is *tiring* physically. After all, why should the body need to sleep at all if it isn't tired?

Lunch should be the main meal of the day – and of course a nourishing one: NO coffee unless decaffeinated. Weak tea (one cup only) is OK, but juices or herb teas are better.

Find time in the afternoon to do the Basic Relaxation Exercise (but don't take a nap). Use a visualization of your choice and choose a mantra to describe how it feels to be blissfully and totally relaxed. Programme yourself to have a good night's sleep that night. Much insomnia is probably the result of habit: if you expect *not* to be able to sleep, you won't. Remember that, for you, your word is always law. Start expecting to sleep well. Remember that energy follows thought, which is how thought manifests in physical reality.

DURING THE EVENING

Start the winding-down process early. If your body has been exercised sufficiently in the course of the day, the only problem remaining is sensory overload and an over-active mind. It is easier to leave a slow-moving vehicle than one that is going at breakneck speed. So take your foot off the accelerator and start to slow down in good time. Don't do anything to stimulate the mind further, such as reading, writing letters, settling household bills and so forth. Any kind of mental strain like studying is definitely OUT if you want to sleep tonight. Watching television is a debatable point: if the programme is light, amusing or visually relaxing (wild-life films, for example) that's fine, but avoid programmes with a lot of action or fast-talking. Horror films and films of violence are a definite 'no-no' for they are disturbing at a very deep level of the psyche. It is far better to listen to music you enjoy.

Try to spend time alone or, if in company, don't get involved in heated discussions or emotional confrontations which will wind you up when you are trying to achieve just the opposite. A session of yoga before the evening meal is good, perhaps followed by a short meditation spent sitting quietly holding a mantra or listening to sounds. It is not wise to meditate just before going to bed, as you will be clear-headed and wide-awake after meditating: it is not one-pointedness you need to cultivate right now, but a kind of 'wooziness' or 'spaciness'.

Needless to say, the evening meal should be light and taken early, without tea or coffee. A glass or two of wine could help the unwinding process if you like.

BEFORE RETIRING FOR THE NIGHT

Take a warm bath by candlelight and use one of the bath oils recommended by aromatherapists, such as lavender or sandalwood. You might like to have background music of a suitably soothing type such as those tapes mentioned in chapter three. Don't have the bath water too hot or stay in for too long. If you want a nightcap, try camomile tea or one of the herbal infusions described below; if you must have your drinking chocolate, make it with half-milk and half-water, since milk can be hard to digest on its own. And do resist any temptation to raid the 'fridge before going to bed!

IN BED
We will assume that the mattress is just right, not too soft or lumpy, and that pillows are the height and firmness or softness that suit you. Lighting also should be to your taste, certainly subdued and perhaps only night-lights. The whole atmosphere of your bedroom should be conducive to relaxation, to escaping from the world – comfortable, snug, secure, like an animal's 'den' where it is safe to curl up and doze off. If that is not so, then high on your priority list should be the intention to make it so. After all, about one-third of the rest of your life is going to be spent in your bedroom! You might like to put on a tape of calming environmental sounds, especially the 'Ocean' tape of the waves: not too loud, but so that you can just hear them as if in the distance, rhythmically ebbing and flowing on to the shore that may evoke your favourite visualization beach. Put on a blindfold and turn off the light (though it may be simpler to do this the other way around!) and relax into the Basic Relaxation Posture. Let your thoughts dwell on only two things: either body sensations or a visualization that is beautiful and calming. Even if you don't doze off right away, no matter; you will be relaxing beautifully and recharging your batteries almost as well as if you were sleeping deeply – in fact, better than if sleep were fitful and shallow.

Alternatives to Tranquillizers

The number of prescriptions for tranquillizers issued in Britain every year has been conservatively estimated at over 20 million. One person in fifty of the adult population is likely to be taking tranquillizers on any day of the year, and 1 in 10 men and 1 in 5 women to be taking them during any twelve-month period. Insomnia could well be one of the side-effects of taking tranquillizers; others include depression, anxiety and, in some cases, addiction. A report by RELEASE in 1982 suggested that more than 100,000 people are addicted to tranquillizers. A further danger is that of overdose: about 4,000 people die every year from drug overdoses. There are signs of growing concern about the over-prescription of drugs, quite apart from the publicity rightly given to the appalling damage done to infants when mothers-to-be take certain drugs during the early months of pregnancy. It is not surprising therefore that there has been a revival of interest in the various alternatives to drugs, encouraged no doubt by the respectability given to some of these 'alternative therapies' by royal approval. So let us consider what they can offer to help handle emotional tension. Broadly speaking, these 'alternative' – or better, 'complementary' – therapies fall into clearly-defined categories:

> nature/herbal remedies
> systems of medicine
> manipulative therapies
> psychotherapies
> self-help therapies

Readers wishing to explore further any of those described below, should contact the addresses given in the Appendix.

Herbal Remedies

Herbs have been used as remedies throughout history and in all civilizations: Ancient Egypt, Mesopotamia, India and China. In Europe the father of medicine, Hippocrates, wrote of the medicinal properties of plants and these were also patiently recorded by monks copying manuscripts throughout the Middle Ages. Our first university, that of Salerno, recommended plant drugs obtainable in the Mediterranean region, while in the early sixteenth century Paracelsus was to write in his *Herbarius* of the abundance of medicinal herbs to be found in his native Germany. In Britain herbalism existed long before the Romans came: the

Druids were experts and their skills survived the Roman occupation to be passed on to the Anglo-Saxons, later to be nurtured by the monks or the lady of the manor caring for her household and estate servants. A best-seller of its time was Nicholas Culpeper's *The English Physitian* (*sic*) published in 1652. Its subtitle probably helped to make it so: 'An astrolo-physical discourse of the vulgar herbs of this nation being a compleat method of physick, whereby a man may preserve his body in health; or cure himself, being sick for three pence charge, with such things onely as they grow in England, they being most fit for English bodies.' Not only patriotic, but macrobiotic to boot! The famous herb garden created twenty years later for the Society of Apothecaries of London is still in existence in Chelsea today (now called the Physic Garden) and has as its aims research into botany and instruction in technical pharmacology with reference to the growing of medicinal plants. Obviously, herbal-ism has a respectable ancestry. It is also undergoing something of a revival, as can be seen from the appearance of herbal remedies on the counters of leading high-street chemists and the research into the healing properties of plants being actively encouraged by the World Health Organization.

Often we enjoy the beneficent properties of herbs to nourish and soothe us as a matter of course. In the kitchen we use parsley, marjoram, dill, rosemary, basil and perhaps alfalfa, a blood purifier rich in nutrients. If we have a cold we may inhale eucalyptus or, if a toothache, desperately apply oil of cloves until we can get to the dentist. Yet some of these herbs are of proven efficacy in calming nerves, lifting depression, restoring vigour and promoting sound sleep – for example marjoram, mint, sage, rosemary and thyme. As an alternative to the camomile tea suggested as a good night-cap for insomniacs, any of these can be tried as an infusion, though mint and lime are the tastiest.

To prepare a herbal infusion is simple. Just pour 1 pint of boiling water over 1 oz of dried herbs or ground root (or half a litre of water to 1 gm herb). Leave for 10 minutes or so to infuse. Drink 1–3 cups a day. They can be sweetened with honey, providing alternatives to those endless cups of tea or coffee full of caffeine. Some insomniacs swear by hot milk with grated nutmeg and a spoon of honey, while in Japan they prefer our remedy for colds: lemon juice, hot water and honey. A cure for insomnia said to date back to the Middle Ages is to stuff your pillow with hops, which also have soothing properties, though this does not sound too comfortable. Rosemary also would do, but that sounds even more uncomfortable! However, nowadays it is not difficult to find herb pillows which are both comfortable and aromatic.

Reference has already been made to the herbs used in aromatherapy. Lavender, sandalwood, cedarwood, jasmine, juniper, rose, orange-blossom and patchouli – all these can be used as oils for baths and massages to soothe and relax tension. Bergamot, another fragrant oil used in aromatherapy, is what gives Earl Grey tea its special flavour.

A word of caution is in place here. As in the case of food supplements, herbal remedies should not be taken over a long period of time, as they build up in the body. Some also have to be treated with circumspection, valerian for example, for doses over a long period could eventually prove toxic. It would be wise to consult a professional herbalist; the training of herbalists in Britain is controlled by the National Institute of Medical Herbalists which conducts a four-year course. A guide to herb suppliers is given in the Appendix.

Bach Flower Remedies

These are remedies prepared from the flowers of wild plants, bushes and trees and they are useful for treating a wide range of sources of emotional tension. In fact the thirty-nine remedies listed below cover every negative state of mind known to mankind (and womankind), so there should be one amongst them that matches your mood. They were the discovery of Dr Edward Bach who after working in London for twenty years as a consultant bacteriologist and homoeopath, gave up his lucrative Harley Street practice in order to devote all his time to finding plant remedies which would heal physical illness – such illness, he believed, being the result of underlying negative emotional states. Since these remedies are not prescribed for physical complaints they are ideal for anybody suffering from emotional tension or undergoing stress, whether or not accompanied by physical symptoms. In times of acute stress the 'Rescue Remedy' (number 39) combining five other remedies is the one that should be used.

THE BACH REMEDIES

1   *Agrimony* For those who suffer considerable inner torture which they try to dissemble behind a façade of cheerfulness.

2   *Aspen* For anxiety, apprehension, fear and foreboding of *unknown* things.

3   *Beech* For those who are critical and intolerant of others. Arrogant.

4   *Centaury* Weakness of will; those who let themselves be exploited or imposed upon – who become subservient and have difficulty in saying 'No'.

5   *Cerato* For those who doubt their own judgement and seek advice of others. Often influenced and misguided.

6   *Cherry Plum* Fear of mental collapse/desperation/loss of control and fear of causing harm. Vicious rages.

7   *Chestnut Bud* The refusal to learn by experience; continual repetition of the same mistakes.

8   *Chicory* The over-possessive who demands respect or attention (selfishness), and likes others to conform to their standards. Those who make martyrs of themselves.

9   *Clematis* For those who are indifferent, inattentive, dreamy, absent-minded. Mental escapists from reality.

10   *Crab Apple* A cleanser. For those feeling unclean or ashamed of ailments. Self-disgust/hatred. Houseproud.

11   *Elm* For temporary feelings of inadequacy; those over-whelmed by responsibilities.

12   *Gentian* For the easily discouraged. Disappointments and *known* depressions.

13   *Gorse* For despair and hopelessness; utter despondency – 'What's the use?'

14   *Heather* People who are obsessed with their own troubles and experiences. Talkative 'bores' – poor listeners.

15   *Holly* For those who are jealous, envious, vengeful and suspicious. And for those who hate.

16   *Honeysuckle* For those with nostalgia and who constantly dwell in the past. Homesickness.

17   *Hornbeam* 'Monday morning' feeling but once started, the

task is usually fulfilled.

18 *Impatiens* Impatience, irritability.

19 *Larch* Despondency due to lack of self-confidence; expectation of failure, so fails to make the attempt. Feels inferior, though has the ability.

20 *Mimulus* The fear of *known* things. Shyness, timidity.

21 *Mustard* Deep gloom or depression that descends for *no known cause* and lifts just as suddenly. Melancholy.

22 *Oak* Brave determined types who struggle on against adversity despite setbacks. Plodders.

23 *Olive* For exhaustion and utter weariness; tiredness both mental and physical.

24 *Pine* Feelings of guilt. Those who blame themselves for the mistakes of others. Feels unworthy.

25 *Red Chestnut* Excessive fear or anxiety for others, especially those held dear.

26 *Rock Rose* Terror, extreme fear or panic.

27 *Rock Water* For those who are hard on themselves – who often overwork. Rigid-minded, self-denying.

28 *Scleranthus* Uncertainty/indecision/vacillation. Fluctuating moods.

29 *Star of Bethlehem* For all kinds of shock, mental or physical.

30 *Sweet Chestnut* The despair of those who have reached the limits of endurance – only oblivion is left.

31 *Vervain* Over-enthusiasm, over-effort; straining. Fanatical and highly-strung. Incensed by injustices.

32 *Vine* Dominating/inflexible/ambitious/tyrannical. Love power and make good leaders.

33 *Walnut* Protection remedy from powerful influences – helps adjustment to any transition or change e.g. puberty, menopause, divorce, new surroundings.

34 *Water Violet* Proud, reserved, sedate types, sometimes 'superior'. Little emotional involvement but reliable/dependable.

35 *White Chestnut* For those with persistent unwanted thoughts. Preoccupations with some worry or episode. Mental arguments.

36 *Wild Oat* Helps to determine one's intended path in life.

37 *Wild Rose* Resignation, apathy. Drifters who accept their lot, making little effort for improvement – lacking ambition.

38   *Willow* Resentment and bitterness with 'not fair' and 'poor me' attitude.
39   *Rescue Remedy* A combination of Cherry Plum, Clematis, Impatiens, Rock Rose and Star of Bethlehem. All-purpose emergency composite for shock, terror, panic, emotional upsets, 'stage fright', examinations, dentistry, etc. Can also be externally applied to burns, bites, sprains and so on.

This use of remedies found in Nature is characteristic of 'alternative' therapies. Also characteristic, whatever the technique used, is a 'holistic' approach: in other words, the healing is addressed to the whole person, not just to the symptoms. This is because the latter are seen to be manifestations of imbalances and distortions of the person's energy, of low vitality and negative patterns of thought and behaviour rather than the result of accidental infection, for example. For those suffering from emotional tension, therefore, they offer much, and certainly more than can be offered by the overworked GP trained solely in the allopathic approach geared to attacking only the manifestations rather than the sources of 'dis-ease', with either drugs or surgery.

Homoeopathy

Homoeopathy must be considered as a branch of medicine peculiarly geared to dealing with stress in its pre-medical forms. There are remedies for excessive tension, fatigue, irritability, compulsive worrying, insomnia – areas in which allopathic medicine has little to offer apart from tranquillizers. Homoeopathic remedies are now appearing (like herbal ones) on the shelves of high-street chemists, but since they are aimed at specific *people* rather than specific *symptoms*, there is no substitute for consulting a practitioner in person. Many of these are qualified doctors (it is well-known that one of H.M. the Queen's physicians is a homoeopathic doctor).

Founded about 200 years ago by a German doctor named Samuel Hahnemann, this quite illogical yet sometimes startlingly effective system of medicine is based on the principle that 'like cures like'. 'Homoeopathy' comes from the Greek words meaning 'similar to the disease', while 'allopathy' (which is what homoeopaths call conventional medicine) means 'different from the disease'. Hahnemann found that a dose of quinine – used to treat malaria – if taken by a healthy person would produce a fever characteristic of malaria. He deduced from this that the symptoms were in fact signs of the body's resistance to the disease rather than of the disease itself. On the basis of this, he formulated the principle that 'like cures like'. In other words, if a harmlessly-diluted dose of a certain poison which produces specific symptoms in a healthy body is administered to someone suffering from symptoms exactly like them, those symptoms will disappear – sometimes very quickly. What makes homoeopathy 'illogical' is that the potencies of the remedies can be so diluted that actually there may be nothing of the original substance left – and still they are effective, more so than in the 'mother tincture' because they have been 'dynamized' in the process of manufacture.

If then the right remedy is found, homoeopathy works: if not, it does not. But at least the wrong remedy will be harmless and, unless taken constantly, will produce no side-efects, which is not always the case with allopathic drugs. There are hundreds of remedies in the homoeopath's reference book, the *Materia Medica*, and the practitioner's delicate task is to find the one that exactly matches not only the declared symptoms of the patient, but a whole constellation of quite subtle energies. Clues are sought in the habits, moods and preferences of the patient; lifestyle and temperament are investigated in an attempt to get the whole picture before a remedy is prescribed in the form of pills, powders, tinctures or ointments. Diagnosis thus obviously takes more time for the homoeopath than for the GP for whom antibiotics, say, may be the obvious prescription for a whole range of conditions.

During a consultation the patient will be encouraged to talk about his or her feelings as specifically as possible as part of the diagnostic process. Sometimes it is a chance remark or a seemingly innocuous fact that provides the decisive clue pointing to 'this' remedy rather than to 'that' one which is similar but not exactly the same. Gabrielle Pinto, a homoeopath and acupuncturist with a successful London practice, was provided with such a clue when treating a recalcitrant case of migraine by the young man's anxiety about his health. Now there are many possible homoeopathic remedies for migraine, but acute anxiety is especially characteristic of poisoning by arsenic. The prescription therefore of *arsenicum album* in the appropriate potency was effective in curing the migraine dramatically. In another case, this time of the allopathically-incurable tinnitus, the all-important clue was the elderly patient's past history of tuberculosis. The unpleasant ringing in the ears that was driving the unfortunate man to distraction was in fact a side-effect of the streptomycin that had been used to treat his tuberculosis. With the prescription of silica a remarkable improvement took place, together with a resurgence of well-being that the patient had not experienced for a long time.

Homoeopathic remedies stimulate the body's capacity to heal itself naturally and their effects continue for a long time – unless, that is, you drink coffee which cancels out the effect straight away. Like acupuncture, homoeopathy is also prophylactic. Many who are taking responsibility for their own health go to alternative health practitioners *before* they get ill, whenever they feel 'down' or 'off' in more subtle ways. These feelings could well be the body's early-warning signals that worse is on its way if attention is not given and changes made to work, diet or life-style. Emotional tension therefore should never be suppressed, or worse may follow. Homoeopathy is available on the National Health Service in London, Bristol, Glasgow and Liverpool and contacts for consultations with qualified practitioners are given in the Appendix. The first consultation is a long one (lasting perhaps a couple of hours) and therefore the fee is usually higher than for subsequent sessions. This is because, in this preliminary consultation, the homoeopath takes time to elicit as much information as possible in order to build up a picture of the patient's whole energy pattern which matches a specific remedy in the *Materia Medica*. No other therapy in existence is more concerned than homoeopathy with the subjective experience of the patient, in pinpointing the exact type of emotional tension, how it feels, when it comes on and a considerable amount of other detail as to the patient's preferences, rhythms and life-style. Whether or not the remedy finally prescribed has any effect (and remember, it has to be 'right on'), one certainly comes away feeling that one has been *seen*, which is therapeutic in itself. Here are a few examples of how answers from a patient to specific questions from a homoeopath help – like pieces of a jigsaw puzzle – to build up a picture of an energy pattern which is then matched against the pattern that goes with a specific remedy.

Overwork, worry, excitement, fatigue. Oversensitive and cries easily. Melancholy and bad-tempered. Nervous, anxious and impatient. Feels cold, especially after anxiety attacks. May wake up screaming during the night. Shy, gloomy, retiring.
Remedy indicated: *Kali Phos*.

Sunk in grief and despair, the picture of 'silent grief'. Sobs frequently. Cannot tolerate contradiction or criticism. Over-sensitive, makes scenes, then distorts what others have said. Unpredictable and irrational swings of mood, sometimes nervous for no reason. Introspective. Tends to blush whatever the emotion. Lack of interest and appetite. Night sweats. Feels burdened in the head.
Remedy indicated: *Ignatia*.

Worried, tired, unable to think clearly. Very critical and suspicious. Hates being alone, yet dislikes company (would prefer to have others within reach). Over-scrupulous, perfectionist. Forgetful. Feels worse in the afternoon. Over-reacts to being thanked or to good news, perhaps by weeping. Hates work and new ventures. Lacks self-confidence.
Remedy indicated: *Lycopodium*.

Physically and mentally exhausted. Anxiety about the future, despair that may border on the suicidal. Thinks often of suicide or death generally. Always discontented, quarrelsome. Sulks; morose and uncommunicative. Poor memory. Feeling of oppression in the chest around the heart; palpitations. Often feels chilled, cold and damp.
Remedy indicated: *Aurum*.

Acupuncture

Used in China for 5,000 years (and still used today), acupuncture is another branch of alternative or complementary medicine that can do something to help those who suffer from chronic emotional tension. Acupuncture was brought to Europe in the nineteenth century by Jesuits who had worked as missionaries in the Far East, where it is used for treating almost everything. At a symposium held by the World Health Organization in Peking in 1979, medical acupuncturists from all over the world compiled a list of diseases which they considered amenable to treatment by acupuncture. There were more than forty: they included asthma, bronchitis, tonsillitis, duodenal ulcers, constipation, diarrhoea, colitis, gastritis, eye disorders, osteoarthritis and the common cold. Among them too were nervous disorders, migraine and toothache, and it has been in the relief of pain that acupuncture has had most publicity in the West. In China it is sometimes used as an alternative to anaesthesia in surgical operations – over 3 million of the latter had been performed by 1979, with no deaths reported. In Munich too, acupuncture has been used in more than 1,500 operations at the German Heart Centre as a way of reducing the drugs administered to anaesthetized patients. In Britain, many National Health Service pain clinics have been using acupuncture on patients with migraines, backaches and so forth which have not responded to drugs or surgery.

Acupuncture, like homoeopathy (and indeed any other more orthodox form of treatment) may not work with everybody, but work it undoubtedly does. *How* it works depends on whether one takes a view from the East or the West. Recent research has suggested that acupuncture relieves pain because it causes the release of endorphins into the spinal fluid. First discovered in 1975, endorphins are chemicals produced by the pituitary gland which have an effect similar to that of morphine in changing mood and relieving pain. They are released during moments of stress, which is why sportsmen or soldiers, for example, sometimes are able to carry on as if nothing has happened when in reality they may have been quite seriously injured. In Sweden, in experiments at Uppsala University, it has been established by professor of pharmacology Lars Terenius that endorphins are indeed released by acupuncture-like stimulation of the body.

Whatever the reason, anyone who suffers from emotional tension, whether or not it is linked with chronic pain, could give acupuncture a try. It is better to consult a qualified acupuncturist rather than a National Health Service GP who may have taken only a short course (sometimes perhaps just a week) in acupuncture and thus inevitably have only a superficial grasp of this subtle discipline. Like homoeopathy, acupuncture seeks to heal ('make whole') the patient on an energy level rather than merely by suppressing symptoms and driving the 'dis-ease' in further; so a similar detailed preliminary investigation is called for before treatment. The acupuncturist's job is to establish where the patient's energy is blocked, stagnating, and to encourage it to flow again through the energy pathways of the body called 'meridians'. There are twelve main meridians, ten of which are associated with particular organs and the other two concerned with circulation and body temperature. According to Taoist medicine, whenever we feel 'off' or under par, energy is not flowing smoothly along these meridians and, if the energy (called 'chi') is not balanced and stimulated to flow smoothly again, we could be in for illness.

Diagnosis of how the vital energy is flowing and of the condition of each organ is by way of looking at the tongue (examining its coating and colour) and by taking the pulse. The latter is a more complex affair than the usual method of just feeling the speed and strength of the blood. The pulse of each meridian, six in each wrist, is felt by pressing lightly or deeply at various points on the radial artery. An experienced acupuncturist will be able to feel as many as twenty-eight different qualities of pulse, which tell which organs are working too hard or too feebly. The points at which needles are inserted (don't worry, they don't hurt – usually!) may have no apparent connection with the part of the body that is in trouble. Migraine, for example, might well call for needling between the big and second toes to treat the liver at the point on the liver meridian called Liver 3. Sometimes, instead of, or together with needles, the acupuncturist may use *moxa*: applying heat to the point by burning a small cone of mugwort and removing the herb before it burns the skin.

Acupuncture then is both prophylactic and healing for those for whom it works. It can relieve pain, soothe the anxious or hyperactive, relieve insomnia and lift depression. Many have also claimed that it has helped them to stop smoking after certain points in the ear have been worked on.

Acupressure

Acupuncture is the domain of the qualified professional and obviously should never be attempted by lay people. With thumbs rather than needles, however, the same points as are used in acupuncture may be stimulated as a kind of first-aid for a whole range of unpleasant conditions. This is called acupressure. It is very simple to apply, can be done anywhere at any time without attracting any attention and is usually effective in relieving tension states, headaches and fatigue – even toothache, temporarily. Pressing firmly on Heart 9 while cringing in the dentist's chair will both prepare you for the assault of his drill and sedate you while the ordeal is under way. Heart 9 is the point at the inside bottom corner of the nail of the little finger. Press the point on the finger of the hand on the same side of the body as the tooth on which the dentist is working.

The technique of acupressure is as follows. Use the tip of the thumb to apply firm pressure – about as much as you would use to make an indentation in a ball of clay. Press for ten seconds, wait for ten seconds and then press again for ten seconds. Don't overdo it and do stop when you feel better. Acupressure should not be applied

- if you have heart trouble
- if you are under drugs or medication
- if you are in the last stages of pregnancy
- after a hot bath
- after eating
- if the point is on an open wound, scar, wart or mole.

The corresponding point on the other side of the body should also be stimulated afterwards. Some useful points are listed below and others will be found by contacting the organizations recommended in the Appendix. To find the point needs a certain amount of preliminary probing, for its exact location varies slightly with everybody – and it must be *exactly* pressed for anything to happen. So don't just press 'somewhere in that area' – find the point itself by probing until you come across a slight indentation and feel a twinge. Then you've got it. Here are some you can practise on.

Hands
    Heart 7 *Anxiety, depression, insomnia, irritability. Sedative.*
    Location in the crease on the side of the wrist nearest to the little finger and in line with it.
    Heart 9 *Exhaustion, irritability. Tonic.* (As for toothache.)
    Heart Constrictor 8 *Exhaustion.*
    On the 'head line' in the palm of the hand below where the middle fingers join.
    Heart Constrictor 9 *Anxiety.*
    Inside the corner of the bottom of the nail of the middle finger.

Legs
    Stomach 36 *General well-being.*
    Below the knee-cap, on the outside of the leg next to the shin-bone.
    Kidney 3 *Nervousness, fear.*
    Midway between the top of the ankle-bone and the Achilles tendon, on the inside.
    Bladder 60 *Anxiety.*
    Midway between the top of the ankle-bone and the Achilles tendon, on the outside.

Feet
    Liver 3 *Tension headaches, irritability.*
    One and a half inches up from the join of the big toe and the second toe.
    (Also: for depression or insomnia, press the middle of the sole of each foot hard, using very firm pressure with the thumb.)

Changing the Energy

What we really want to happen when we are tense, irritable,

anxious or depressed is to feel good again: in other words, to move out of a negative energy-state into a more positive one where we are relaxed, happy, at ease with ourselves and the world. So far in this chapter we have considered ways in which our mood will be changed by boosting our energy by treatment 'from the outside': with vitamins, herbs, homoeopathic remedies, acupuncture and acupressure. Let us consider now how we can also change the energy 'from the inside' and lift ourselves out of troughs of habitual tension, irritability or despondency. Provided that we really do want to drop our negativity and not to wallow in it, to play victim and to manipulate others, there is much we can do for ourselves.

AUTO-SUGGESTION

Auto-suggestion as a technique for reviving energy in the body has already been discussed. It is also a powerful tool for changing moods. Feelings are generated by thoughts much of the time and, provided these feelings have not been given too much energy by brooding on them, it is often possible to change the energy-pattern simply by changing the thought-pattern. But one has to give up wanting to be *right* in favour of wanting to feel *good* again. You are of course free to hang on to negative thoughts as long as you wish. But if you are aware of what they do to you and what experiences they attract, then you will come to realize that you are cutting off your nose to spite your face. You have to ask yourself whether it really is worth killing yourself to get attention or sympathy by playing weak, harassed or helpless, risking a stroke by winning an argument or suicide by continuing to wallow in depression or resentment.

Emile Coué, the father of modern hypnotherapy, was careful to emphasize the importance of stimulating the creative imagination to bring about positive attitudes rather than forcing them through will-power. He advocated yoga and the use of mantras to quieten the mind as a preparation for instilling the seeds of these positive attitudes through affirmations, themselves a form of mantra. Coué's best-known affirmation was 'Every day, in every way, I am getting better and better,' to be repeated with total concentration each day, morning and evening. The advantage of this one is that it covers a multitude of sins because it is so general. Here are some more specific ones that could be used when we feel we are building up to a row or a sulk, a black depression or simply another grey day.

Unspecific tension/irritability

'I feel totally relaxed, contented, at peace with the world.'
For those 'Monday morning blues': 'Today is going to be a beautiful day. I'm going to enjoy everything that happens.'

Specific worries

'All is well, and all manner of things shall be well.'
Remind yourself that you have had worries before and *still* you are here.
Remember how you worried then and now you have forgotten it all; it is finished, gone.
Ask yourself: what is the very worst thing that can happen. So what?
Allow yourself to make a mistake, to be an ordinary, imperfect human being.
(Note: It is not suggested that one should be entirely passive and resigned if a worry is obsessive: if something *can* be done, do it.)
Perhaps it is totally appropriate to be worried: there may indeed be a threat imminent which can be averted by action. But when all that can be done has been done (or if there is nothing to be done) then worrying is just losing energy and should be dealt with like any other unproductive emotional tension. In that case, the only way to stop worrying is to *drop* worrying.

Nervousness, performance anxiety

'I feel full of confidence . . . totally confident and relaxed.'
'I am going to really relax into this performance and enjoy it.'

As with auto-suggestions aimed at fatigue, these can be combined with or followed by visualizations designed to get into the body the *feeling* of ease, confidence, relief from worry etc. Before leaving for an important interview, for example, imagine in some detail the actual interview in progress, the questions that are likely to be asked by the interviewer or the panel; see yourself answering with ease, grace (and perhaps humour), their being obviously impressed with you, the final offer of the job or whatever it was you were being interviewed for. See the news being relayed to you. Does it come by letter, a phone call? Enjoy the sweet smell of success in your visualization and establish the feeling in your body that it has actually happened already. See yourself sharing the good news with your family and friends and receiving their warm congratulations. Open a bottle of champagne: one of the nice things about visualizations is that no expense may be spared! Rather than allow worry to keep you tossing and turning all night, calm yourself down with the Basic Relaxation Exercise, then visualize that the object of your worry has resolved itself in the most favourable way possible. What is the best thing that could possibly happen? Create it in your mind's video, setting the scene with attention to detail, rehearsing the dialogue and directing the action and bringing your home movie to the happiest possible ending. The most important things to go for in these visualizations are detail and getting the feeling of release from tension into the body. Whatever happens subsequently, positive thinking can bring only good things, from helping you to relax. Energy is freed as you expand instead of contract; others respond to your positive attitude; your performance will be more relaxed.

MEDITATION

Sitting in meditation, silent and still, watching thoughts come and go, serves to bring peace of mind by distancing us from the objects of aversion and desire that disturb it. We come to realize that 'This too shall pass', so why take it so seriously? As they say in zen:

> sitting quietly,
> doing nothing,
> the grass grows by itself.

By and by the turmoil of thoughts settles down, like mud that has been stirred up from the bottom of a pond by constant probing with a stick. The best way to let the mud settle, to gain clarity again, is simply to relax, to wait and see what happens. At first, if one is very tense, this may not be easy. But with practice, watching the breaths and focusing on the hara, regular meditation allows us to slip out of 'this world of sound and fury' into calmer spaces from which we can return refreshed and clear, the better to handle real situations that may be causing tension.

'Meditating on the opposite' should be tried whenever we have so much going on with us that 'just sitting' is out of the question for the moment. It is a form of meditation 'with seed' (i.e. content) rather than the meditation 'without seed' which is just sitting, empty, watching. As such it has something in common with the techniques used in autosuggestion already described and is just as powerful in changing energy and mood. It consists simply of letting the thoughts dwell on the *opposite* of what you are feeling right now. Since you are feeling emotionally tense, the opposite will therefore be a positive and relaxing emotion. For example, whenever you are feeling nervous, try focusing your thoughts on 'confidence': let your mind wander to the times when you really did have confidence in yourself, how it felt then. Conjure up images of people you know who do have this quality of self-assurance; see them in action handling their affairs and relationships with quiet assurance; imagine yourself in their place. If your problem is loneliness, dwell on 'friendship' or 'togetherness'. Meditate on what is the nature of friendship, conjure up the faces of people you have loved. Consider how isolation is really a myth, how everything and everyone in this world is interdependent, how it all interacts to foster life and change. Don't confuse alone-ness with loneliness; you don't have to feel lonely just because at this moment you find yourself temporarily without others around you.

If you are feeling angry with someone or generally irritable, practise the beautiful Buddhist meditation called 'metta', 'loving-kindness'. This meditation consists simply in putting out gentle, loving energy to all beings and everything in the Universe, without any exception. Of course, at first you won't feel at all loving because your reality is that you are in a bad mood – which is precisely why you should practise this meditation, to exchange that reality for another. And why not change it? After all, what else are you going to do with your anger? Dump it on someone else? Turn it inwards, sulk and make yourself miserable? Pretend it is not there, repress the energy so that it makes you physically ill?

Instead of brooding over your wrongs and feeding this bad mood (which you will have to come out of *sometime* anyway) decide to drop it. Withdraw energy (i.e. attention) from who said/did what to whom and generally playing 'ain't it awful?' and put energy rather into regaining your peace of mind. This is not the same as repressing or pushing down anger: what you have chosen to do is to direct the anger energy into another channel, which is not at all the same thing. And energy is energy, pure and simple: there is no such thing as sex energy, this energy or that energy. Anger and compassion are two sides of the same coin, two aspects of the same vital force. So as you sit in meditation, breathe in patience and forgiveness, breathe out negativity and violence – and include forgiving yourself if you feel neither patient nor forgiving for a while. Be at peace with the world. Is it really all that bad? Think of the love and caring that is shown to you every day that perhaps you don't even notice, let alone how Life sustains you. Visualizing loving-kindness as a light may help: let it bathe first of all the people you like. As you calm down, extend it to those you don't like and wish them well. After all, they are human beings like you, sharing this tiny planet somewhere in the vast universe: you have much in common. Then gradually, let the light of your goodwill radiate out to all those brothers and sisters out there, living their lives in the only way they know how, this vast family you have, some of them happy, some of them living in hell – and wish only good things for all of them.

By now all the tenseness and contraction that goes with negativity will have dispersed; you will feel expanded, calm, at peace with yourself again.

LETTING OFF STEAM

'A trouble shared is a trouble halved,' they say. Whoever THEY are, they are right for several reasons. It comes naturally to us to turn to a sympathetic listener whenever we feel upset or uptight, for we know instinctively that it will make us feel better. We may not so much need advice as a chance to unburden ourselves of our feelings by sharing them. Just allowing ourselves to be open, authentic with another human being is of itself healing and soothing and this was probably the original appeal of 'going to confession' in the Catholic church. What we may receive from the friend in whom we choose to confide our worries and fears is, however, not absolution and exhortations to righteousness (unless we are unlucky), so much as another viewpoint. If we are *very* lucky, we may even come away not taking everything quite so seriously if our friend has laced humour with sympathy and a willingness to listen non-judgmentally.

Sometimes, too, in sharing our tale of woe we may be encouraged to actually express strong feelings rather than to keep a 'stiff upper lip'. This catharsis, 'letting off steam', is the quickest single way of discharging the energy contained in pent-up feeling. It is also one of the hardest things to do in our modern society, which by and large disapproves of the direct expression of strong feelings and conditions us to repress them, at least in public. But what makes for a more 'civilized' society on the outside makes also for considerable emotional tension at a personal level – and a lot of mental and physical illness as well. It is an axiom of physics that energy cannot be destroyed, only transformed. We have seen that, provided we are not too upset, techniques like 'meditating on the opposite', autogenics, changing breathing and so forth will work to move us into calmer spaces. But sometimes we may feel totally untogether, off-centre, furious, paranoid or grief-stricken and then the energy is too much for us to handle on our own. 'Dumping' our stuff indiscriminately is no good: it will only alienate, antagonize or bore others. Repression on the other hand is equally bad: anger lingers on as resentment, grudges and sulks, while fear turns into anxiety. A definite correlation has been established between undischarged grief and illness, while other repressed feelings may host a whole range of illnesses of the skin, bones, circulatory, digestive and respiratory systems, not to mention acute depression or other mental illness. At the very least, we don't feel good with what the founder of Gestalt therapy, Fritz Perls, called 'unfinished business' – unresolved tension.

Structures do of course exist within which catharsis is possible, even encouraged, either on a one-to-one basis or within groups. Psychotherapy no longer carries either the mystique or the stigma it once had, but it can work out expensively, especially on a long-term basis. Occasional counselling and support in times of stress is available on the National Health Service and addresses are given in the Appendix for anyone who feels temporarily unable to cope with what is happening in their lives. The approach used by the therapist will vary, but what is essential is to be listened to non-judgmentally and allowed to go into the feelings which are proving hard to handle. *Understanding* what is happening will, with luck, come later. More important is to *experience* fully what is happening, to give yourself permission to own to whatever feelings there are and to go into them. During the seventies, group therapy became fashionable, but this popularity has suffered a decline in the eighties and there are few 'Growth Centres' around to offer the primal, encounter and bioenergetic groups where people could really let off steam. In such groups participants would be encouraged by the group leader to be authentically self-expressive: bodywork, inter-personal confrontation and a whole battery of techniques would be used to take the lid off suppressed feelings. People would beat cushions with their fists (or a tennis racket) and wring a towel to death until they were exhausted in order to purge their anger. Violent, yes, and disturbing to some; but at least they were discharging negative energy harmlessly instead of harming others or turning it in on themselves.

If strangling a towel or beating a cushion is repugnant to you, hard exercise could do the trick in changing negative energy states. Running is particularly good, or chopping logs. Any sport where you have to *hit* something will also discharge emotional tension – squash or tennis, for example. The important thing is to really *use* your body energy to the utmost. Sometimes, in fact, emotional tension is simply the result of not using one's body sufficiently, of being immobile too long or inward looking for long periods. Swimming is good, not least of all because the water will help to clear your energy field of negativity. Provided it is expressive and total and not just a token shuffle, dancing is an excellent mood-changer and harmonizes body, heart and mind energies. However you decide to do it, find some way in which you can 'let off steam' harmlessly. You will be providing yourself with a safety-valve and will feel a whole lot calmer afterwards.

EMOTIONAL STRESS RELEASE

Try this technique if there is something stressful or disturbing that you simply cannot get out of your mind.

Sit in an armchair or at a table on which you can rest your elbows. Place the tips of the fingers on the forehead, lightly touching the bony bulges, and keep them there throughout this exercise. Only touch with sufficient pressure to prevent your fingers slipping off the brow as you stretch the skin a few millimetres towards the hairline.

Concentrate now on whatever it is that is bothering you. Let your attention dwell on the situation, recalling the harsh words perhaps, and the distressing scenes that are still painful to remember. No matter how painful this may be or how upsetting, as long as you keep your fingertips on the forehead the pain, distress and hurt will just melt away. Suspend disbelief and just try it. It is impossible for anyone to remain emotionally upset whilst doing this, and the amazing thing is that the calming effect is permanent. The problem will never trouble you again to the same extent. Give yourself enough time to really *feel* the feelings that you are deliberately recalling and stop when you feel finished.

FOCUSING

To get rid of tension arising from 'unfinished business', it is important to work through the feelings still lurking under the surface which are causing that tension. As Werner Erhard, founder of est (Erhard Seminar Training) puts it: 'Whatever you resist, persists. Whatever you experience totally, disappears.' Often we resist experiencing unpleasant feelings, afraid that we will be swamped by them or that we may act on them and get ourselves into trouble. Yet acting out negativity will not be necessary (though you will still have the choice) if you give yourself space to really *experience* your anger, jealousy, despair or whatever it is that is ruining your peace of mind.

In case you are still unconvinced that it could be that simple, try this focusing exercise. Tune in to what is going on with you right *now* at this very moment. What are you feeling, *exactly*? Give a name to that feeling. Try to label it very specifically, catching its *nuances* as finely as you can. Keep zoning in on exactly what you are experiencing at a feeling level from moment to moment – and keep labelling. You will find that as soon as you have successfully 'caught' (i.e. experienced) a feeling, it changes into something else. Paradoxically too, the willingness to experience *whatever* is real for you right now brings relief and distance.

PRAYER

In times of great stress, many people who would not normally consider themselves 'religious', who only find themselves in a church at christenings, weddings or funerals, resort to prayer as an outlet for unbearable tension. Many millions all over the world also pray regularly as a normal part of their daily lives and no doubt draw strength and inspiration from so doing. It would of course be impertinent to discuss the validity of prayer as such in a book intended as a guide to relaxation, and even to suggest its efficacy for this purpose will probably be seen as irreverent by those with faith in it and irrelevant by those without. I still recall being quite shocked in my earnest Catholic schooldays by a Jesuit father telling us that 'Prayer doesn't change God – it changes *us*.' This definitely smacked of heresy to me and I regarded him with deep suspicion for the rest of that upper school retreat.

Yet, quite apart from whether there is actually 'Anyone Up There' to hear and respond to our prayer, it certainly has the power to transform our experience of reality (i.e. to change our energy-state), provided it is heartfelt and trusting. In view of what we have discussed so far as conducive to dissipating emotional tension, it is not hard to see why. To begin with, prayer can be a form of sharing one's pain, perplexity, grief, anxiety and of asking for support. It can be a focusing of thought forms on the positive and a clarifying of what we really would like to be the case – for a loved one to get well again, for example, or for strength or clarity to see one through a difficult time. At the very least, prayer thus mobilizes inner resources of energy in a very positive way while also taking us deeper into the actual experience of what is real for us right now – a form of focusing. The actual physical structure that goes with some forms of prayer enhances the relaxing effect: withdrawing to a quiet place (a chapel?), kneeling (yoga or meditation posture?), candlelight, soft organ music (sense relaxation), eyes closed (sense withdrawal?), repeating invocations (mantras?), reciting the rosary (worry beads?) etc.

Yet the effects of prayer go far deeper into the unconscious, activating the great archetypes of the human race and tapping into their healing energy: the Saviour, the Great Mother, the Divine Child. Jung found that in most of his patients in middle age and after, their problem was a religious one, of finding meaning and direction in their lives. He also postulated in his *Modern Man in Search of a Soul* that the atrophy of the religious function in the modern psyche has nowadays cut most people off from feeling connected with Life and of 'in-touchness' with the deeper levels of the psyche, expressed in the symbols and rituals of religious forms in every culture. That this energy can be destructive is only too obvious in the world today where so much slaughter is being perpetrated in the name of religion, whether Christian, Moslem, Judaic, Hindu or Buddhist. 'Men will wrangle for religion; write for it; fight for it; anything but – live for it.' (Colton) On a personal level, too, half-baked religion can make us miserable and guilty or drive us crazy. But it is also true that, for very many, prayer and faith do help them to cope with the tensions of modern living and above all, with *change*. For change is about Time and Death and unless we have worked out some way of including change in our philosophy of life, emotional tension will be more difficult to handle when things start slipping away from us and 'ain't what they used to be' – looks, power, prestige, health, potency . . . Surrendering to what is the case instead of fighting it is relaxing, and 'Thy Will Be Done' the most relaxing of all mantras.

NON-SERIOUSNESS

Laughter is the best medicine of all for emotional tension. It is indeed a natural way to discharge tension, as in the tense expectancy artfully built up in an audience by the professional funny-man. When he finally delivers the punch-line we fall about laughing – and enjoy doing so. The essence of all problems is *seriousness*, which is what makes them so heavy. If you can get to see the funny side of any situation, it ceases to be a problem.

Everything is as serious as we choose to make it, including Death itself. There is a story from Old China about three friends who were clowns. They used to travel from village to village just making people laugh with their zany antics and total irreverence. For years they travelled together through the countryside and wherever they went they were welcomed, for they helped the poor to forget for a while their problems and their poverty and cheered them up no end. One day, staying in a village in a Northern Province, one of the clowns died during the night. Next evening, after a day toiling in the fields, the villagers gathered around the funeral pyre to watch the body being cremated. 'Now,' they said to each other, 'for the first time we shall see these fellows sad, for they have lost their dear friend.' They stood in respectful silence when the remaining two emerged from a hut bearing the heavily shrouded body of their friend and placed it gently, lovingly on the pyre. There was a hushed silence as the pyre was lit and the flames began to lick the corpse's shroud. Suddenly the villagers nearly jumped out of their skins at a succession of loud bangs. Firecrackers concealed in the dead man's shroud exploded in rapid succession and rockets shot up into the night sky, showering into streamers of coloured light. Wide-eyed, startled, holding their sides with glee, all enjoyed this splendid send-off, grateful for the entertainment and to the dead man for going out 'with a bang'. The two clowns were laughing too, albeit with tears in their eyes. And (who knows) maybe their friend's spirit was laughing too. Sometimes it is the only thing we *can* do.

CHAPTER SEVEN

Getting Out of the Rut

Once upon a time there was an Emperor of China who thought he was dying, so weak, listless and depressed was he. Nothing pleased him any more and his advisers and physicians, unable to come up with any cure for his malaise, feared for their lives as the Emperor became more and more irritable every day. They scoured the land for anyone who might help them to heal their master and restore him to good spirits. They were overjoyed when one day a Taoist sage turned up at the court claiming to have just the right remedy for the Emperor's disease. 'There is,' he said to the ill-tempered Emperor, 'a precious stone in your garden which will restore you. It is a magic gem and buried deep. Find it, and you will be well again.' The Emperor immediately started to give orders, but the impassive old man cut him short. 'No sir, others can not do it for you, for only you can find it.'

Grudgingly, the Emperor heaved himself out of the bed from which he had not moved for weeks, called for a spade, and accompanied by the sage and curious counsellors, headed for the garden which surrounded the palace. They eventually came to a halt at the spot indicated by the sage. 'Here,' he said, 'is where you have to dig. Remember, the stone is buried deep.' The Emperor set to work. Day one passed with him puffing and blowing with the unaccustomed effort – but without unearthing the stone. Day two passed in the same way, the Emperor by now almost invisible in the deep hole but clearly audible as he cursed the sage and threatened execution if he proved to be lying. That night the Emperor's snores could be heard throughout the palace as he slept more deeply than ever before in his life. On the third day his guards were startled early in the morning when he cheerfully called for a hearty breakfast and then set off, humming to himself, to resume his digging. By now the hole was very deep and from it the astonished courtiers heard the recently moribund Emperor singing to himself as he dug away. Relieved, they summoned the sage and asked him how long it would be before their master found the precious stone. 'Sounds like he's found it already', was the answer. But by now the Emperor (who was no fool) had also got the message. 'Who needs a stone?' he laughed at the end of the day. 'Thanks to that old rascal, I've never felt better in my life. He shall be rewarded!'

Up to this point, we have seen how to recharge our batteries and how to avoid getting drained by losing energy. But the reason for energy not flowing may be because it is stagnating rather than because it is insufficient, and if this is the case, we will feel just as 'down', fatigued, listless and unsatisfied.

IS THIS YOU?
'I don't know what's the matter with me. I do nothing all day and I'm always tired.'
'I'm so bored at work I could scream. Same old routine, day in, day out.'
'Our relationship is very stuck. We just don't have anything to say to each other any more.'
'I've always wanted to . . . (move to the country, get out of this business, take the Trans-Siberia Express, etc. etc.) but of course it's just not possible because . . . (I'm too old, there's so much unemployment, I don't have the money etc. etc.).' (What's *your* excuse?)
'Everyone else always seems to be having more fun than me (to be better off, living more fully, doing more with their lives etc. etc.). But then, I never had the opportunities they had . . .'

Moving Energy

When energy is stuck, the first thing to do is to move it in any way you can. Sometimes, as in the case of the Emperor, merely taking some unaccustomed exercise will recharge us with energy. After all, we get the energy we need: if we are too laid back, too lazy, we don't need energy. We put on weight, our muscles get flabby and the more we sleep, the more we want to sleep. Exercise not only gets us back into the body and moves its energy, it also refreshes the brain and body cells with oxygen and thus livens us up. What exercise and how much to take is up to you – and of course it goes without saying that one should not be too drastic in changing old habits too fast. Jogging is fashionable at the moment, while aerobics seem on the way out. Running has become quite a cult, with marathons and sponsored events. (When before in the history of the cinema could a film about *running* have won Oscars as did *Chariots of Fire*?) Anyone bored with ball-games could get a kick of a different kind by learning one of the martial arts, which also have the advantage of centring one's energy. And if all this sounds too much like hard work, you could always just take a walk in the park or with the dog. For the really lazy, a couple of sessions with an acupuncturist could also move your energy out of the rut.

Freshness

The direct opposite of feeling in a rut is the experience of *freshness*. This is the quality that children have, but which adults have lost – except when they go on holiday. For when we go away on vacation, we tend indeed to 'become as little children' again, which is why we have such a good time. At least, that is what happens if we are not forced back into our adult selves by having to cope with problems like hotels over-booking, lost passports or similar nightmares. Consider exactly what it is that makes for that 'holiday feeling', when we feel life is so good we wish it could always be like this and we didn't have to go back to the old routine again. Cast your mind back to that holiday when you had such a good time . . . What did you do? How did you feel then? Do a focusing exercise/visualization and recapture that elusive 'holiday feeling' again. *This* is freshness, this is what we mean by 'quality' in our lives.

Freshness is a quality which we have to work on – or, rather, to invite into our lives – for the natural tendency of everything is to grow old and stale. Reflect now on how you created the 'holiday feeling' for yourself with a view to perhaps recreating it on a rainy day in London when you are back at work again, suntanned and wistful, nostalgic for those lizard days on the beach and those balmy nights wining and dining *al fresco* or dancing under the stars . . . Of course, your idea of a holiday may be completely different: pony-trekking, bird-watching, yachting, touring archaeological sites or whatever turns you on. But the essential ingredients of the satisfaction generated in you could well include some or all of the following.

Changing your usual routine

'A change is as good as a rest' – a cliché, but often true. Habit dulls.

Open-ness to the new

New places, new faces. The unfamiliar is *interesting* and energy follows interest – quite the opposite with boredom. The more unfamiliar the people, territory, language, customs, the more stimulation we get.

Contact with Nature

Enjoying beautiful scenery, lakes, mountains, sunsets at sea – these refresh our senses and remind us what a magical world this can be if only we have eyes to see. Its grandeur too can fill us with something akin to religious awe as we contemplate the spectacular and timeless . . .

'Coming to our senses'

Not only seeing afresh, but refreshing the other senses with new sounds, of the markets, *souks* and *medinas* perhaps, or of music played on bazoukis, mandolins, sitars . . . The fragrance of unfamiliar flowers, or of fresh-caught sea-food being delivered to restaurants from whose kitchens a variety of mouth-watering smells is being wafted . . .

Trying out the local specialities, sometimes disappointing but rarely boring, lingering over those drinks that we would never dream of buying at home even if they were obtainable there, we literally savour the new.

Exercise, Body-awareness
The Chinese Emperor felt much more alive simply because he got back into his body and used it again. When on holiday we use our bodies or become more aware of them, thus both relaxing and moving energy at the same time. We explore our new surroundings, swim, expose our bodies to the sun and air or climb, ski, surf . . . As well as feeling good, we put energy into looking good also with our lotions and oils for sun and after-sun, attention to dressing appropriately for whatever activity we shall be enjoying that morning, afternoon or evening . . .

Intention to enjoy
The attitude we take with us on holiday has a lot to do with our experience of it. If we expect everything to go wrong, most likely it will. More often, however, we expect to have a good time and, unless we are unaware or unlucky, we do. We are geared for enjoyment, looking around for things to enjoy. Some people of course do just the reverse: they are always looking around for things to complain about, but then if they enjoy complaining they are enjoying in their own way anyway. *Intend* to enjoy and you will.

Absence of pressure
The delicious sense of freedom we get from 'being away from it all' has much to do with the absence of pressure. It's off for a while and there is nothing we *have* to do. There are no alarm clocks, no rushing off to work in the morning, no housework or cooking (unless we are camping, but then it's fun and everybody mucks in). Not only is the daily grind suspended, but we experience *choice*: how we choose to spend the day is entirely up to us. We have no one to please but ourselves. We have given ourselves space to be at source rather than reacting to outside pressures – which is another way of saying we can do *what* we like *when* we like.

We may not always be in this blissful position of being able to do what we like whenever we like: most of us have a living to earn, family and other responsibilities. Neither can we be always on holiday. But what we can and should do is to take a holiday whenever we can afford the time and the money, and especially when life starts to look grey. If this is not possible, then at least we can try to recapture that holiday feeling. Here's how:

- Do something new every day – something you have never done before. Anything to break up the old routine will do, even if it is as simple as taking a different route to work or buying a newspaper you don't normally read.
- Commune with Nature whenever you can and in any way you can, even if it's only sitting or working in the back garden. Try to get away for a weekend to the country or the sea. Go for walks, take a picnic, enjoy . . .
- Try to get away for the weekend anyway, anywhere to have a change of scene.
- Take more exercise. Get yourself massaged. Go for a sauna. Get into your body more.
- Give yourself more space to be alone with your thoughts. Use the focusing technique or meditate to get more in touch with yourself and what you need to create in your life right now in order to experience satisfaction.
- Drop a few of the more oppressive structures in your life. Say 'No' to a few of the people who have expectations of you.
- Be totally selfish for a while and spoil yourself. Give yourself treats you wouldn't normally do. Be totally hedonistic and playful.
- Clean up your living space and make it beautiful. Change the furniture around to make it even more pleasing and comfortable.
- Go out and buy yourself new clothes – if you can afford it, a completely new outfit. Have your hair done and, if you feel adventurous enough, change your image.
- Start being less goal-oriented. Or rather, don't make *things* your goal rather than the quality of your life. You may have to turn down money and job offers in order to give yourself more leisure time to do what *you* really want to do.
- Be more creative, more imaginative in the use of your leisure time. Instead of doing the same old, tired things, venture into new spheres. Cultivate new interests and hobbies just for their intrinsic interest. Start doing things, not to *get* anywhere, but just for *fun*.

Creative Leisure

As well as creating leisure in life, it is important to use that leisure creatively. This does not necessarily imply actually *making* things, although going to pottery classes, for example, could well be right up your street as a way to channel your energy. Rather, it means using free time to balance the one-sidedness of having to work for a living. For the greater part of most days, most of us are functioning in a certain mode. The mode in question depends on the type of job we do. For example, academics will be working with ideas and words, articulating concepts, being *logical* – in other words, in their heads all day. Others will be exercising their capacity for *caring* – nurses, for example, and social workers. For some, it is *decision-making* that earns their bread and having to choose between alternative policies, while for others what their job entails above all is very fine *attention to detail* and extreme accuracy. For those in a managerial capacity it is *organizing and controlling* staff and schedules – quite the opposite of those who are paid for *receiving and obeying orders*.

To misquote William of Wykeham, 'Habits maketh man' and each job brings its own bad habits – or what the French call its *déformation professionelle*. What is appropriate within the work context is not necessarily so outside it and can be a pain in the neck for others who have to live with it, whether it is the intolerance of contradiction of the schoolteacher, the bossiness of the managing director, the nitpicking of the logician or even the social conscience of the welfare worker. These people are 'on' twenty-four hours a day, and unable to switch off. Identification with their jobs makes them not only boring but less than human, for human beings are many-sided and their 'job side' is only one aspect. If it is prestigious or currently trendy they may well hide behind it; if not, they may be apologetic about being under-achievers. Either way they are stuck with being what they do for a living, which of course turns them into *things*. Feeling in a rut is the experience of stuckness and to get out of it is to create experiences for yourself that make you feel what in fact you are – a free human being and not a thing.

The essence of freedom is having a choice. Giving yourself more and more *choice* in your life frees you from old habits, structures, outside pressures – and raises your energy. So whenever you feel jaded, bored, trapped (all manifestations of 'rutness') an antidote is to start making a few choices, preferably of things that you have never tried before. Choose to exercise parts of you that are not nourished by your work. Most commonly it is the left side of the brain that works overtime and the right side that is under-developed in the course of the day. Left-side brain deals with logic, language, detail, 'getting things done'; right-side brain with feeling, sensing, intuiting, sensuality. We need them both and we need *balance* if we are not to become either aridly intellectual and worldly or over-sensitive and other-worldly. If you feel 'something is missing' in your life it is almost certainly this: that your life is too one-sided – and probably left-sided. Here are some of the leisure activities and interests that might do the trick in balancing up such one-sidedness. The list is only intended to give you a few ideas and maybe to strike a spark – it is not suggested that you do them all!

Right side brain 'stimulators' for those whose rut is about feeling too much in their heads, arid, routine-bound, over-structured and organized:

  music
  literature and poetry
  visual arts, theatre, cinema
  meditation
  yoga
  martial arts
  travel (though not the organizing side – leave this to others!)
  therapy/growth/conscious-raising groups
  contact with Nature
  communication at a feeling level with people you love and trust
  surrender – to anything or anyone (but choose wisely!)

Left side brain 'stimulators' for those who feel spacy and unconnected, uncreative, blocked and too introverted, isolated:

  crafts
  language study
  academic courses of study
  organizing anything
  planning and detailed work

writing
sport
exercise

Some activities draw on both sides of the brain in that they need both acquisition of technique, concentration and feeling, e.g. painting or playing an instrument.

Choosing not to be a Victim

We have seen that low energy states go with contraction, high energy with expansion, *expansiveness*. Whenever we are under pressure we feel hemmed in, shut off from what we would really like to be doing by having to do what we feel we are expected to do. Energy does not flow freely into tasks unwillingly accepted: they are experienced as chores to be done for fear, favour or money. On the other hand, when we have freely *chosen* to do something, we tend to put our energy into it; instead of dragging reluctantly, we can actually get 'high' off the challenge and the effort involved, plus feeling satisfaction at the end from attaining the goal we have set ourselves.

Playing victim is just about the biggest rut one can get into and it is very common. Every day one hears the 'victims' complaining: about their work, their wives, husbands, lovers, the weather. For victims, it is *always* either too hot or too cold, it wasn't their fault – and the other person is always wrong. To be around someone who is always complaining is one of the surest ways to become drained; understandably so, for the complainers are unwittingly draining themselves by losing energy to negativity and thus need to gain energy from others. This is called 'leeching' or 'sucking': like leeches, they will suck you dry if you let them, bleeding you until you are as drained and lifeless as they are. There is no way to get high with somebody playing life-games like 'Ain't It Awful?' and 'Poor Me!' Try to jolly them into a better space and they will fall back on the counter-ploy of, 'Yes, but . . .' Victims have an answer for everything, and very plausible answers they are too. And they are right: looked at through *their* eyes, that's the way the world is. But then, looked at through *anybody's* eyes, that's the way the world is, for there are as many worlds as there are people. We all create our own experience of the world and select the facts to validate this experience. What makes a victim a victim is that he or she is unaware they are *choosing* to see the world in such a way as to make them feel like victims.

How are you *not* to feel a victim, contracted, helpless, hopeless and low in energy? Simply by reminding yourself that you always have *choice*, by ceasing to blame and by taking back the responsibility for your life – and with it, your power. Blaming others is castrating for them and, less obviously, for the blamer also. How do they come to have power over your life and who gave it to them? Others in fact have as much power as you choose to give them. Whatever the circumstances (which you probably set up anyway, either by making the wrong choices somewhere along the line or by abdicating your power to choose), what you make of them, how you interpret them is mostly up to *you*. As Richard Lovelace wrote to Althea from his prison in the seventeenth century:

> Stone walls do not a prison make,
> Nor iron bars a cage.

There is a beautiful story in zen of the old man who returned home to his village hut and surprised a robber making off with what he had managed to steal while the old man was out. To the robber's amazement, the old man called him back to help load up more loot, with the words: 'You poor thing, you must be poorer than me to be so desperate. Here, take the lot, you obviously need it more than me!' This old Buddhist is like the Christian who 'turns the other cheek', returns hate with love and perhaps the shirt off his back too – they are refusing to be victims and thus keeping their inner freedom. What happens is what happens: what *you* make of what happens is the experience you get from it.

Try Changing Your Attitude

Usually, whenever one feels in a rut and that life is getting drearier and more predictable by the day, the obvious thing seems to be to seek *outer* change. Sometimes it will work, and some of the ways in which this could be done have already been suggested. But sometimes it will not work and we merely take our negative attitudes and staleness with us on holiday and feel just as fed up in foreign parts as we were at home. If we have moved house or changed jobs, we are likely to find the same snooty or intrusive neighbours (perhaps with noisy kids) or the same abrasive work conditions as before. If we have changed partners very likely we may well have leapt out of the frying pan into the fire and be playing the same destructive games with each other all over again. We take ourselves with us wherever we go. So before chucking it all in and moving on to a new job or relationship, see first if you can change the outer by changing the inner – in other words, changing your attitude to whatever it is that makes you feel you are in a rut.

- *Stop blaming and take responsibility*
  You are where you are now as a result of saying 'Yes' or not saying 'No'.
- *Take back your power*
  If you are willing to admit you said 'Yes' you admit to the power to say 'No', to switch energy from playing victim into transforming or changing your situation.
- *Be clear as to what you want*
  Take space to tune in to exactly *how* you are in a rut. What is missing in the quality of your life? Use focusing and visualization techniques to bring the vague discontent into focus.
- *Set yourself goals*
  Write them down: short-term goals and long-term goals. Make them realistic *and* don't limit yourself. Pin up the list of goals in your room and look at them night and morning to remind yourself of the direction you have established in your life.
- *Drop the past*
  By 'past' is meant all the old habits of thinking and reacting that have created and perpetuate the rut you feel in. They may include: values, 'certainties', ways of relating, self-image, resentments, grudges, games, manipulations – and the satisfaction of complaining and nagging! Choose to let go of them, even if it hurts, in order to allow freshness and more quality into your life.

- *Stay in the present*
  Don't assume that because Life seemed a drag yesterday (half an hour ago?) it is going to feel that way NOW. Open your eyes to what is going on around you this minute – it is always fresh and new, a situation you have never experienced before. Listen to what your partner is saying and reach out to him or her. Respond rather than react, which is what you will do naturally if you 'lose your mind and come to your senses'.
- *Stay positive*
  This does not mean repressing 'down' feelings, but refusing to be *brought* down by them. You are not your body, your feelings or your thoughts, but the one who experiences them. Don't let others bring you down either. A soft answer turning away wrath is not being weak: it is refusing to allow somebody else's negativity into your own space or to get angry just because *they* happen to be angry. Choose how *you* want to feel – and if you want high energy, stay positive.

To Move or Not to Move?

Working to change your attitude rather than your surroundings often does the trick and gets you out of your rut. Putting *more* energy into the job that you find boring, for example, or more love into the relationship that seems dead – transforming duty into service and habit into intimacy – could fan life out of the ashes at work or at home. But if, having tried this, you still feel dissatisfied, unfulfilled and restless, then perhaps it is time to move on. First, however, it is necessary to take stock, to look before you leap lest at some later date you regret what you have left behind.

This restlessness, this dissatisfaction, could well be a sign that there is more within you that is wanting expression, more creativity, more depth of relating. Life is wanting you to move on – and not to heed its call is to invite at best increasing deadness and frustration and at worst depression and possibly physical illness. Somebody I know has been complaining recently about how boring his job is, yet he cannot summon up the courage to leave a job that at least is *secure*. Not surprisingly his health has been suffering, for he is a very gifted and creative person. The new energies wanting to be manifested in the world are turning destructive for want of expression and will eventually force him to stop slogging away at a daily grind that is wearing him down. His problem is a common one: how to have challenge and freshness *and* security. Alas, they do not seem to go together; one has to settle for one or the other and it would appear that many have opted for security and as a result have stopped really *living*.

Use the focusing and visualization techniques described earlier to establish contact with whatever it is that you need right now in your life. Try to pinpoint exactly what is missing, what would 'deliver the goods' in terms of freshness, stimulation, satisfaction. See yourself in the future – contented, happy, full of life and enthusiasm: What are you doing? Who are you with? Where are you living and what sort of life-style are you following? When you start looking inside yourself and asking these existential questions, you are likely to come up with answers in your dreams. Be interested in these dreams and see them as statements of your life-situation, pointing in the direction where your energies want to take you. Keep a notebook by your bed and write down any dream you may remember on awakening, before the memory fades. Recall the dream at intervals during the day and try to feel its message rather than endeavouring to analyse it intellectually.

Taking Risks

We have suggested in earlier chapters that life provides us with the energy we need to meet its challenges. However, if we play safe and shirk these challenges, the reverse is true: energy stagnates and we become deader and deader. Excitement and security just do not go together and we have to choose whether we want a comfortable grave (be it a 'safe' job or a boring but predictable relationship) or whether we want to feel truly alive. It is precisely for this reason that many people engage in hair-raising pastimes just for the hell of it, so as to get high off the adrenalin that flows when one takes risks, when the outcome is not certain. Probably this, rather than greed, is the reason why so many people gamble. Whenever we feel ourselves to be in a rut, it is a sure sign that life is too predictable, too 'safe', and that perhaps we need to take more risks, to raise our sights, to be a little more ambitious or more open to new possibilities. The mere fact that we feel discontented is a good sign: it means that a part of us is still alive and wanting to experience more, to *be* more, to express and create more. What usually militates against this alive and adventurous part is the 'dead wood' – fear of moving into the unknown, fear of change. We rationalize this other part of us that wants to play safe, that is fearful, with reasonable-sounding excuses such as, 'I'm too old to move/change.' If this is indeed the case, then we may as well give up living, for if life is anything it is Change – changing energy manifesting in changing forms. Change we must, either in the form of continued growth and movement or in the form of decay and death. And one is never 'too old', as anyone who has successfully weathered the male or female menopause will know. Too old for what? Doing the same old tired things, perhaps, but for living and growing – never. There is always more, but we have to drop the past to allow in the new. And the real risk is in trusting that if we follow where the energy wants to take us, that Existence will support us. This has certainly been my experience time and time again: leaving an outwardly successful but stultifying teaching career after fifteen years to travel the world; settling in India to learn yoga and meditation; returning to the West to establish a business and to enjoy the good life again (by 'good' is meant 'comfortable' – India is not the most comfortable place in the world!); getting bored with just making money and then training to be a psychotherapist; writing books because that was the next thing that I wanted to do . . .

Significant changes in life-style will always be attended by *angst*, uncertainty as to whether one is doing the right thing and probably warnings of doom from one's friends, who rarely want us to change and who feel as threatened as we do by the unknown. But every effort made to get ourselves out of a rut will generate energy and freshness for us. We feel more alive and it is better to have tried and failed than never to have tried at all! And the more we risk and succeed, the easier it becomes to move on, as we learn to trust our feelings about what we need to be doing with our lives.

Keep on Growing

The way to stay young, fresh and full of zest for living is to keep on growing – whatever your biological age. Some people are old in their thirties and forties: stuck, bored, tired and stale. Others seem to have found the elixir of youth even when they have passed retiring age. They stay enthusiastic and interested in what is going on around them, their energy is high and positive, they enjoy life and remain curious about what it is going to bring them next. It is this willingness to explore the 'more' that life has to offer in the way of experience that is the real elixir. Far from killing the cat, curiosity keeps it lively and kittenish.

Personal growth is about self-awareness and open-ness to new experience. It is about learning the ways of the world and one's own ways of relating to that world, about energy and its laws and how to live in harmony with them to avoid having a bad time. It is about getting to know who one is and what one needs to be happy, where true creativity (vocation?) lies and how to transform weaknesses into strengths. It is about more and more acceptance of oneself 'warts and all' and increasing one's ability to tolerate real intimacy with others, and to do with one's own vulnerability, transparence and authenticity. There is so much to learn about life: it is vast, multi-dimensional, kaleidoscopic. It is willingness to go on learning that keeps humans young and fresh. There is a zen saying: 'Zen mind, beginner's mind' and if zen can be said to be *about* anything, it's about freshness. To think there is nothing to learn is to admit to being in the biggest rut there is.

In the beginning, effort is needed to get ourselves out of any rut, either to move into a different job, environment or relationship or, first, to try seeing them with different eyes. The enemy is habit, routine, staleness, settling for security rather than going for quality in life. Courage is needed to make changes or, failing that, desperation. It helps to get support and one of the small miracles that start happening when you begin moving in the direction that life wants to lead you, is that support does start to manifest. As they say in India: 'When the disciple is ready, the guru appears.' By 'disciple' is meant 'someone ready to learn' and 'guru' means a friend who has learned a thing or two and is willing to share it with you and guide you a few more steps on the way. Your guru may turn out not to be a teacher: he, she or it could be a chance acquaintance, a book that starts you thinking along new lines, a lover . . . virtually anything or anyone who jolts you into a new awareness, a new direction.

For those interested in exploring their potential for living more fully, there are a variety of groups, workshops, seminars and training courses geared to personal growth which have been developed in the human potential movement over the last twenty years or so. They vary from high-powered American imports like est and Silva Mind Control, through gestalt, transactional analysis and psychosynthesis to women's and relationships groups. A technique called Voice Dialogue has recently arrived in this country from America; this is ideally geared to any of us who feel stuck in any way, whether in boredom, workaholism or depression. Developed by ex-Jungian analyst Dr Hal Stone, Voice Dialogue restores to us the power to harness and harmonize the different energies within us which can drain us if they are in conflict and can drive us to distraction and exhaustion if we allow them to control us. Working with a Voice Dialogue facilitator, one comes to recognize these different parts or 'voices' within us: the Workaholic, for example, and the Perfectionist who never wants us to slow down or relax our efforts; the Child (often a vulnerable Child) who would like to play truant from work and just have a good time; the stern Controller who keeps us tense and uptight in case we enjoy ourselves too much . . . Getting to know these parts of ourselves gives us more insight into *why* we do what we do and also puts us in touch with our real needs – essential if we are to avoid losing energy and getting run down, fatigued and emotionally tense and frustrated. Respecting these parts but not allowing ourselves to be controlled and manipulated by them, gives us more freedom and choice in our lives – and that means more quality. It is beyond the scope of this book to discuss these avenues of growth further and the interested reader should refer to the contact addresses listed in the Appendix.

CHAPTER EIGHT

How to Replenish Your Energy

(This chapter is a resumé of what has already been discussed in the previous chapters and should prove a useful reminder of what you can do whenever you feel that things are getting on top of you).

Fatigue and tension are energy phenomena and the results of either:
Losing energy and getting drained (by stress, rushing, overdoing, over-commitment, emotional tension, sensory overload etc.) **and not recharging our batteries** (by poor nutrition and digestion, not enough sleep, relaxation, rest periods/time off) **or stagnating** (not enough fresh air, exercise, stimulation and change etc.).

FATIGUE/TENSION SYNDROME	RELAXATION SYNDROME
controlling	allowing
tensed muscles	let-go
locked-in posture	open posture
shallow breathing	slow, deep breathing
contracted, 'uptight'	expanded, expansive
under pressure	feeling one's space
compulsive thinking	slowed down thought process
negative feelings	feeling good
physical discomfort	at ease
sensory overload	soothing environment
seriousness	enjoying, playful
energy in head	body awareness, sensuality
low or scattered energy	energy accumulating, centred

TEN GOLDEN RULES FOR REPLENISHING YOUR ENERGY
  1 *Be more sensitive to your energy levels*: Warning signs that you need to ease up and nourish yourself:

irritability, pessimism, depression, inability to unwind, muscular aches (especially shoulders, lower back, neck), eyestrain, headaches, sleep disturbances (insomnia, waking up very early, feeling unrefreshed on awakening), listlessness, feeling there is no time for anything, constant indigestion, obsessive worrying, rushing when there is no need, exhaustion, pains or tightness in chest.

2 *Slow down*: breathe slower and more deeply

slow down movements, e.g. walk more slowly, give yourself more time to do things

talk only when you have to for a while

do only what really needs to be done right now

cut down on your commitments

don't over-structure your time (and that includes leisure)

take breaks as often as you can and as soon as you start to experience strain (if only a visit to the wash-room!)

3 *Feel your body again*: body awareness *is* relaxation. Become aware of it in any way that is practical at the time, for example:

stretching

opening up the posture (uncrossing legs, straightening back etc.)

self-massage (head, hands and neck should be possible in most places; feet in some)

bathing

receiving massage

yoga

exercise

4 *Switch off*: get enough sleep and make sure you sleep well.

learn sense-withdrawal

practise the Basic Relaxation Exercise every day

use a mantra

use auto-suggestion

use visualizations

5 *Nourish your body*: in emergencies use the stress diet and take supplements, especially vitamin B complex, vitamins C and E, calcium lactate or calcium pantothenate (for tension) and ginseng (for energy). Cut out junk food, drugs and stimulants. Include enough protein, fresh vegetables and fruit, whole

grains and fibre in your everyday diet. Cut down on salt, sugar and foods high in cholesterol. Don't skip meals, but fast occasionally or go on a cleansing diet. Pay proper attention to the preparation of your food and *how* you eat.

6 *Refresh your spirit*: create a harmonious and relaxing aura in your living (and if you can your working) environment, giving attention to colours, lighting, pictures etc.

learn to enjoy silence, stillness, solitude; sometimes practise regular meditation

stay in contact with Nature any way you can, both indoors and out

get more into 'right-side brain' activities (e.g. music)

stay open to the new

make space for the non-goal oriented – have *fun*

7 *Stay positive*: negativity drains you, brings you down. Don't cling on to your negative feelings: choose either to share them with a view to work through them (not at all the same as 'dumping'), transform the energy – or just drop them, using meditation on the opposite

focusing

stress release technique

visualizations

affirmations (for a more positive self-image)

'alternative therapies' (homoeopathy, acupuncture/acupressure, herbalism, Bach remedies etc.)

8 *Put the quality of your life first*: bring awareness to your priorities, especially the ones implicit in your life-style of which you may be unaware, e.g. work/money comes first. Give some thought to what you want out of life, whether you are getting it – and if not, why not?

9 *Stay in charge of your life*: however much you may feel at times a victim, remind yourself that we are all responsible for creating our own experience. So take back your power to change whatever needs to be changed, to get the experience of living that you want. Drop the past, set realistic goals for the future – and keep on growing and learning who you are.

10 *Your own special way of replenishing your energy is . . .*
You may already have discovered a way to unwind and

recharge your batteries quickly that has not been mentioned so far in this book. If not, keep on searching, as people have been searching throughout the ages, for in the process you will stay in tune with your process and learn the ways of energy. The Ancient Romans had their Baths, just as modern Californians have their hot tubs. The Athenians (a cultured lot) used to enjoy a night out at the theatre *al fresco* just like today's Londoners or New Yorkers (but with the stars, alas, only on stage). The insights of the East into the laws of Tao, chi, prana (i.e. energy) have come up with the healing and martial arts, meditation, zen and yoga (though your modern Indian is less likely to be found relaxing on his head than glued to film or TV screen or participating in what must be the noisiest festivals in the world). Fatigue and tension are everybody's problem and always have been – and that includes kings as well as commoners – and we all have to find our own ways of beating it, of relaxing and refreshing ourselves in the way that suits our temperament best. For Catherine the Great it was having her feet tickled with a feather and discussing philosophy; for her rival Frederick the Great, writing history and poetry. Louis XIV's hobby was supervising the building of Versailles, while his cousin Charles II preferred stud-farming. When the cares of state got too much for her, Elizabeth I would play the virginals, whereas the second Elizabeth is more likely to have recourse to homoeopathy. The more energy you have to put out in the course of your working day, the more imperative it is to know how to get it back, to nourish yourself. The bigger the star, the greater the risk of burning out too soon, as has been seen tragically so often in show business. So when one reads in the gossip columns that Linda Evans grows orchids at home, or that Elizabeth Taylor likes to have an aquarium in her theatre dressing-room, one gives these ladies full marks for being on the right lines by thus bringing Nature into their space. We may not all be stars, but we do all need to be careful not to burn ourselves out.

Appendix

For the readers who would like to explore further, the following contact addresses may prove useful.

Allergy and Environmental Medicine Department
Nightingale Hospital,
19 Lisson Grove,
London NW1 6SJ

Association for Humanistic Psychology in Britain
62 Southwark Bridge Road,
London SE1 0AU
Tel: 01-928 8284

For a list of therapists specializing in therapies like Gestalt, Transactional Analysis, Bioenergetics etc.

British Acupuncture Association
34 Alderney Street,
London SW1 4EV
Tel: 01-834 1012

For a register of members.

The Society of Homoeopaths
11a Bampton Street,
Tiverton
Devon EX16 6HH

For a list of all homoeopathic doctors and hospitals in Britain.

British Tai Chi Chuan Association
7 Upper Wimpole Street,
London W1M 7TD
Tel: 01-935 8444

Tai chi, originally one of the martial arts, is now primarily practised for its power to centre and to calm. Set sequences of movements are carried out in slow motion with total concentration. It looks both weird and graceful – and is a powerful meditation. The Association teaches it.

British Wheel of Yoga
General Secretary,
80 Leckhampton Road,
Cheltenham,
Glos.

For a list of all the qualified teachers of yoga throughout the country. Your local education authority will also have details of evening classes.

Centre For Autogenic Training
15 Fitzroy Square,
London W1.
Tel: 01-388 1007

Group and individual tuition.

CRUSE (The National Organisation for the Widowed and their Children)
126 Sheen Road,
Richmond,
Surrey.
Tel: 01-940 4818

For support when under stress from bereavement.

Dr Edward Bach Centre
Mount Vernon,
Sotwell,
Oxon OX10 0PZ
Tel: 0491 39489

For all information regarding the flower remedies and supplies.

Mysteries
9 Monmouth Street,
Covent Garden,
London WC2
Tel: 01-240 3688

For 'Ocean' and other visualization tapes.

Relaxation For Living
Dunesk,
29 Burwood Park Road,
Walton-on-Thames,
Surrey, KT12 5LH
Tel: 09322 27826

A registered charity, Relaxation For Living aims are 'to promote the teaching of physical relaxation to combat the stress, strain, anxiety and tension of modern life and to reduce fatigue'. Day and evening classes in courses of 6 or 7 at weekly intervals. Leaflets and tapes.

Shiatsu Society
3 Elia Street,
London N1
Tel: 01-278 6783

For a list of all practitioners in the UK.

Touch For Health Foundation
Brian Butler,
39 Browns Road,
Surbiton,
Surrey.
Tel: 01-399 3215

Provides training courses and workshops in Applied Kinesiology.

Traditional Acupuncture Society
11 Grange Park,
Stratford-upon-Avon,
Warwicks CV37 6XH

For a register of all graduates.

Vegetarian Society
53 Marloes Road,
London W8 6LA
Tel: 01-937 7739

For cookery lessons and lectures.

Voice Dialogue
Sheila Borges,
P.O. Box 22,
London SW17 0HA.

For details of training workshops and a list of facilitators (including the author).

Westminster Pastoral Foundation
23 Kensington Square,
London W8 5HN
Tel: 01-937 6956

Confidential individual and group counselling for personal, marital and family problems. A contribution is expected but nobody is denied help through lack of money. Telephone for an appointment and ask for the Intake Secretary, weekdays 9.30–4.30.

Herbal Suppliers
Neal's Yard Apothecary,
Neal's Yard,
Covent Garden,
London WC2.
Tel: 01-379 7222

Culpeper,
21 Bruton Street,
London W1.
Tel: 01-499 2406
(Culpeper shops are to be found in nine towns in the UK, three in London).

Mail order stockists:
Culpeper,
Handstock Road,
Linton,
Cambs CB1 6NU.
Tel: 0223 891196

Index